Total Fitness the NBA Way

Other NBA books from HarperCollins

Six Times As Sweet
NBA 1997–98 Rookie Experience
WNBA: A Celebration
Official NBA Trivia

Published by HarperEntertainment

Total

Fitness

the NBA Way

The Official NBA Workout Guide for Athletes and Weekend Warriors, from the Experts Who Train the Pros

Timm Boyle

HarperEntertainment
An Imprint of HarperCollinsPublishers

All photography property of NBA Photos. Individual photography credits as follows:

Cover (Abdur-Rahim): Andrew D. Bernstein. **Cover (Smith):** Jesse Garrabrant. **Cover (Iverson):** Kent Smith. 4: Steve Babineau. 32, 41, 76, 121: Bill Baptist. ix, 3, 15, 36 (Fox), 39, 73, 89, 91, 94, 111: Andrew D. Bernstein. 24 (Christie), 36 (Phills), 46, 48, 51, 55, 64, 68, 81, 87, 101, 125: Nathaniel S. Butler. 35, 50: Scott Cunningham. 24 (Mutombo): Tim DeFrisco. 8: Gary Dineen. 109: Garrett Ellwood. 22, 28 (Starks): D. Clarke Evans. 61, 72, 95, 106: Sam Forencich. 1, 12, 13, 14, 16, 17, 18, 19, 20, 25, 42, 43, 53, 54, 56, 57 (Smith), 58, 59, 62, 63: Jesse Garrabrant. 34, 71, 114, 129: Barry Gossage. 49: Don Grayston. 31: Andy Hayt. 30: John Hayt. 29: Ron Hoskins. 52, 67: Glenn James. 6, 23, 27, 83: Fernando Medina. 115: Peter Reed Miller. 37: Jennifer Pottheiser. 122: Jeff Reinking. 11, 44, 118: David Sherman. 38: Kent Smith. 104: Norm Trotman. 112: Ron Turenne. 21: Scott Wachter. 7, 28 (Malone), 33, 45, 57 (Mason), 85, 93, 96, 99, 107: Rocky Widner. 74: Steve Woltmann. 65, 97, 102, 120: NBA Photo Library.

HarperCollins books may be purchased for educational, business, or sales promotional use. For information please write:
Special Markets
Department, HarperCollins Publishers Inc.,
10 East 53rd Street,
New York, NY 10022–5299.
FIRST EDITION
Designed by Pisaza Design Studio, Inc.

Library of Congress Cataloging-in-Publication Data
Boyle, Timm.
Total fitness the NBA way: the official workout for athletes and weekend warriors/ Timm Boyle.— 1st ed.
    p. cm.
Includes bibliographical references.
ISBN 0-06-107303-2
Physical fitness. 2. Exercise. I. Title.

GV481.B68 2000
613.7'1—dc21

99-049024

00 01 02 03 04◆10 9 8 7 6 5 4 3 2 1

I dedicate this book with love and appreciation to my wonderful father, William, who left us for a better place during 1999, and to my daughter, Kaitlyn, who entered this world several months later and has brought us so much joy; to my loving wife, Deanna, and my incredible mother, Jeanne; and to my terrific stepsons, Jon and Tyler.

Contents

Acknowledgments ix

Foreword x

Introduction xii

1. Stretching and Flexibility 1

2. Aerobic and Cardiovascular 21

3. Strength Training and Weights 46

4. The Care and Prevention of Athletic Injuries 65

5. Nutrition 103

References 126

Acknowledgments

Brian Silverman is one of many people who helped make this book a reality. His vision steered this project through some rough waters and brought the book to its final form. I also want to acknowledge the entire athletic training community. These healthcare warriors have an often thankless job, but their professionalism and dedication to serving athletes is invaluable. They do so much more to keep athletes healthy and competing at full strength than most sports fans will ever know. I especially want to thank the four NBA athletic trainers who took part in this project—Tom Abdenour of the Golden State Warriors, Roger Hinds of the Dallas Mavericks, Ed Lacerte of the Boston Celtics and Chris Tucker of the Atlanta Hawks—as well as Rich Dalatri, assistant coach and strength & training coordinator of the New Jersey Nets.

Finally, I owe a debt of gratitude to my sister, Carol, and my brothers, Bill and Dave, for their encouragement throughout the process of writing this book.

Foreword

My career as a player in the NBA lasted for fifteen years and there is no question in my mind that proper stretching techniques, and strength and conditioning programs, were huge factors in the longevity and success I achieved. Not only did I have few injuries throughout my fifteen years in the league, the ones that I did have, I recovered from very quickly. In my twenty-seven years as an NBA head coach, I have always put the utmost importance on proper conditioning and fitness. I believe that there is a strong correlation between the overall fitness of a team and that team's success. And anyone who takes the time to condition their body will succeed at a much higher rate even if they are not full-time athletes and only weekend warriors.

In preparing your body to meet the challenges of competition through strength and conditioning programs, you will also need sound stretching techniques and proper nutritional guidelines. The combination of strength training, conditioning, stretching, and proper nutrition, will help you to perform at a higher level with fewer injuries. Those four ingredients, along with information on the care and prevention of injuries are all covered in detail in this book, *Total Fitness the NBA Way*.

Total Fitness the NBA Way is brought to you by the trainers and coaches who make it their business to get some of the top athletes in the world, the players of the NBA, into peak physical condition. They are experts in their field and the advice and training programs covered within this book will work for both serious athletes, as well as for those just trying to improve their overall physical condition. There is valuable knowledge here if you want to use it.

There is just no substitute for being in top condition.

Lenny Wilkens
Head Coach
Atlanta Hawks

Lenny Wilkens holds the career record for most wins as an NBA coach. He has been selected to the Hall of Fame both as a player and as a coach. He is also the author of Wilkens Legacy Basketball Clinic Series: The Basics. For information about the series log on to www.wilkenslegacy.com.

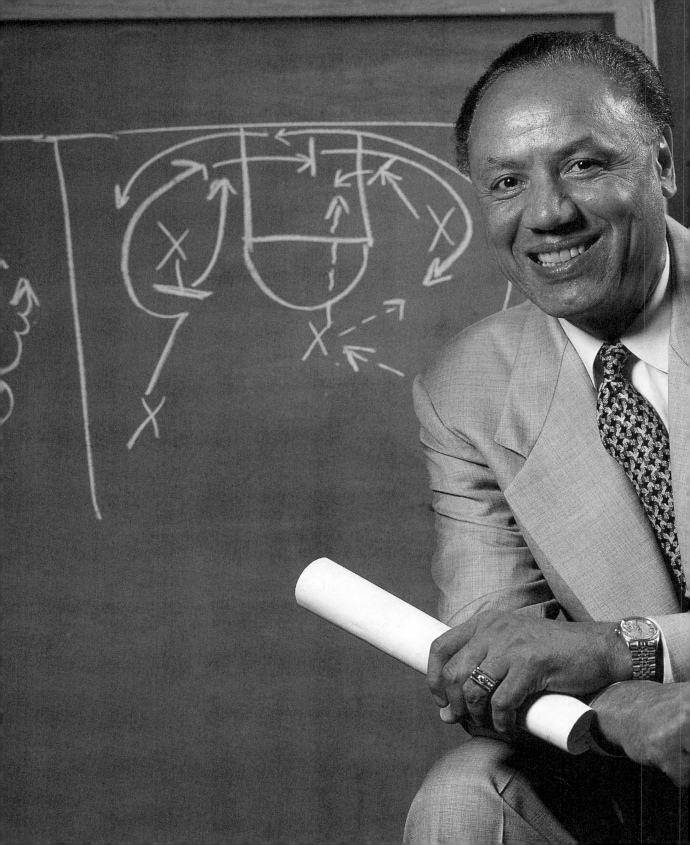

Have you ever tried to play a game of pickup basketball with only three or four players on your team? If you're up against a five-player team, you're probably going to have a tough time staying competitive.

Well, the same is true when you are not at a level of fitness that will allow you to perform at your best. Unless you get involved in a well-rounded fitness program, you're going to be imbalanced. If you're an athlete, it doesn't do much good to have a strong upper body but tire quickly, or to have a great cardiovascular system but be inflexible. You won't realize the full benefits of a stretching program if you don't eat right, and even a good diet won't help you avoid injuries.

Just as a good NBA team needs talent at five distinct positions—point guard, shooting guard, small forward, power forward, and center—your body requires five individual fitness components to stay in shape and enable you to maximize your potential as an athlete. Those five important areas of fitness—Stretching and Flexibility, Aerobic and Cardiovascular, Strength Training and Weights, Care and Prevention of Injuries, and Nutrition—are the titles of the five chapters in this book.

The National Basketball Association is made up of some of the best conditioned athletes in the world, and a lot of them got that way through the influence of the men whose insights and input made this book possible. Among those who made significant contributions to this book are NBA head athletic trainers Ed Lacerte of the Boston Celtics, Chris Tucker of the Atlanta Hawks, Tom Abdenour of the Golden State Warriors, and Roger Hinds of the Dallas Mavericks, as well as New Jersey Nets assistant coach and strength and training coordinator Rich Dalatri.

Because this book is endorsed by the NBA, many of the photos, illustrations, and examples focus on NBA players. But you don't have to be a basketball player to benefit from reading this book. Whether your sport is football, baseball, hockey, soccer, volleyball, tennis, lacrosse, or one of many others, this book's guidelines for getting into shape and staying there apply to you as much as they do to those who spend most of their recreational time on the basketball court.

Following are some of the ways you can benefit from reading this book:

- The **Stretching and Flexibility** chapter tells you not only how this facet of fitness works, it also teaches you specific stretching exercises that will help increase your range of motion and improve your overall coordination.

- The **Aerobic and Cardiovascular** chapter describes how lowering your resting heart rate through aerobic exercise helps your overall health, and it provides you with fitness training circuits that the pros use.

- The **Strength Training and Weights** chapter gives you an insider's look at how certain NBA players have taken their game to another level with weight training, and it offers you the specific exercises that can make it happen for you.

- The **Care and Prevention of Athletic Injuries** chapter shows you not only how to avoid certain common injuries, but also informs you how the pros return to the court quickly and safely from injuries through effective rehab methods.

- The **Nutrition** chapter explains why certain foods are good for you and others aren't, and it supplies you with the breakfasts and pregame meals that an NBA athletic trainer recommends to his players.

So, don't get caught shorthanded on the basketball court or any other playing field. Learn how to incorporate all five components of fitness into your life in order to become a better athlete and a healthier person.

Note: Before beginning this, or any other training program, see your physician for a physical so he can rule out any possible medical problems that might result from the exercises prescribed in the following chapters.

—Timm Boyle

Chapter 1

Stretching and Flexibility

Stretching exercises were a mandatory part of the practice regimen, but one of the role players on this particular NBA team consistently refused to participate. The athletic trainer, a stern look on his face, would admonish the player and preach to him that stretching was a vital part of preparing himself to be successful. The player, however, was a guard whose specialty was long-range shooting. When he came into the game, it was usually to start jacking up three-pointers in an effort to create instant offense. So the player saw no need to spend fifteen or twenty minutes stretching before each practice.

"Hey, listen," the player told the trainer. "You don't need to stretch to shoot."

STEVE SMITH

1

Ed Lacerte has heard it before. In fact, Lacerte, who is in his thirteenth year as the head trainer for the Boston Celtics, has a secret to tell. "Larry Bird will admit that he did not spend enough time stretching early in his career," Lacerte says of the Celtics Hall of Famer. "Eventually, he considered it extremely helpful. But you also have to remember that he was in tremendous physical condition."

The player referred to earlier, whose name is not even worth mentioning, ultimately hurt himself by avoiding stretching, and his NBA career lasted fewer than three hundred games. Who knows? Perhaps his attitude toward stretching mirrored his attitude toward physical fitness in general and eventually led to a premature retirement. While someone as talented as Larry Bird may be able to overcome a casual approach to one part of fitness, a player competing for a roster spot has no such luxury. The old bromide holds true among players who win the last three or four positions on a team: It is truly survival of the fittest.

"I've known athletes who would just kind of hang out," says Lacerte. "Sure they could play, and a lot of them were very good, but who knows how good they could have been if they had maximized their potential?"

Like the journeyman, the casual athlete also needs the extra edge provided by a good stretching program. "Weight training and nutrition have received a great deal of emphasis in recent years," Lacerte says, "but flexibility is still an overlooked, frequently misunderstood and controversial area of fitness for many athletes and coaches. An athlete's performance is directly connected to the capacity of his muscles to move through a wide range of motions."

If you have never spent time stretching, and the task of beginning a program seems daunting, Lacerte says, well, relax. "The good news for athletes, including recreational athletes who have fallen out of shape, is that you can regain flexibility by establishing and following through on a proper stretching program. The more often you stretch, the easier it becomes, and it's much less difficult to maintain flexibility than it is to gain it back after losing it."

Why is stretching important? There are many reasons, technical and practical, but to name a few: It serves as a

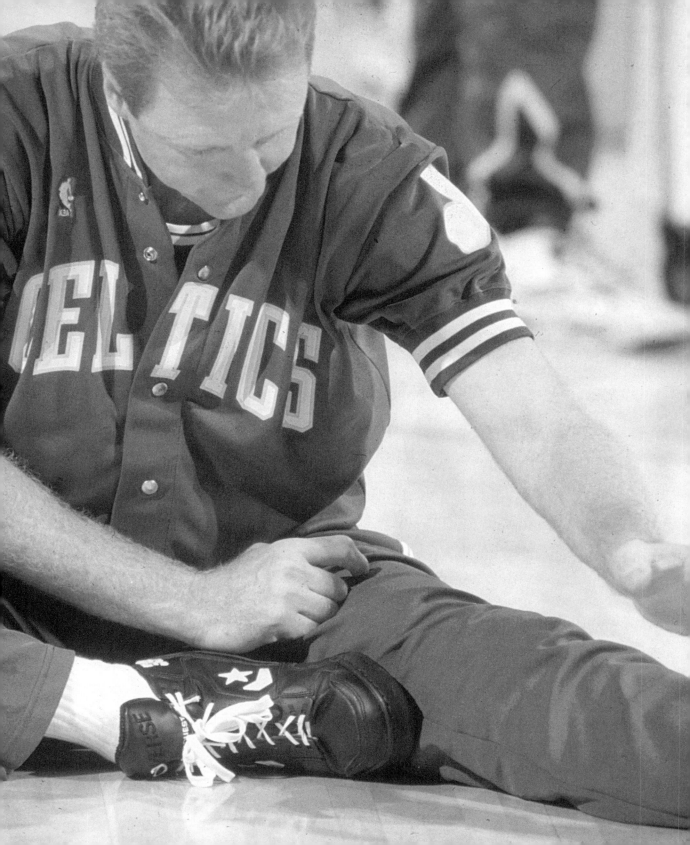

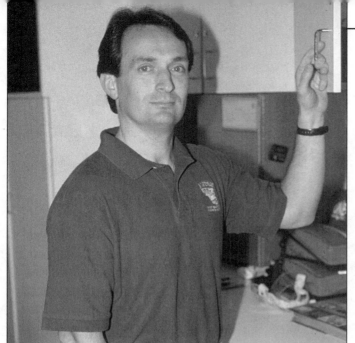

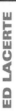

good warm-up for other exercises. It helps you mentally prepare for the coming activity. It helps with coordination. It reduces muscle tension. It helps increase performance. It decreases the chances of injury. And, conversely, if you don't stretch, it can put you at an athletic disadvantage with your peer group. "I know every kid who plays basketball doesn't spend the time stretching that he should. The guys in the playground or the gym, they just go out and play," says Lacerte. "But if they did spend some time on it, they would find that it would help their overall performance."

So how much should the non-professional athlete stretch? Very simple. "Every day," Lacerte says, "regardless of whether you're working out or competing that day. The longer that muscles go without being stretched, the stiffer they'll become and the more difficult it will be to stretch them out again."

A variety of stretching exercises are provided later in this chapter. Lacerte recommends several types of stretches. Some call for holding stretches for twenty to thirty seconds, while others emphasize a range of movement. Lacerte also says that it is important to have a complete stretching program that includes stretching after a workout or competition.

"Most experts agree that pre- and post-workout and competition stretching is vital," he says. "Workouts and games can seriously test the elasticity of your muscles, so a warm-up to increase the temperature of your tissues followed by a systematic stretching routine will prepare those muscles for the rigors ahead. Stretch again after your activity because your muscles will probably never be warmer than they are immediately following a workout or competition."

One thing Lacerte believes strongly is that it does not matter what your age or your level of competition, or whether or not you are just a shooter. Stretching helps to improve your performance.

"Stretching to achieve or maintain flexibility is important to athletes at all levels," he says. "But it also represents an extremely important transition phase for occasional athletes interested in reaching the next level of their athletic pursuits. It's also especially important to athletes who are getting up in years or are out of shape. The more often you stretch, the easier it becomes."

As with the other fitness components highlighted in this book—aerobic and cardiovascular, strength training, nutrition, and injury prevention—flexibility is only one aspect of overall athletic fitness and should not be overemphasized. Controlling your movements by weaving flexibility and strength together is the key to athletic performance.

The Benefits of Stretching

Sure, you want to get right out on that court, but take the extra time to warm up . . . it will definitely be worth your while. Here are some reasons why:

- You will experience a dramatic increase in your range of motion.
- Your performance, including more speed and power and improved muscle recovery, will increase.
- You will perform a skill in its entirety and with greater ease.
- You will reduce muscle tension and experience a more relaxed feeling.
- You will have better coordination.
- You will become more mentally prepared for the upcoming activity.
- You will increase your body awareness because you will focus on the areas you are stretching.
- You will decrease your chance of injuries.

My Body Is My Business

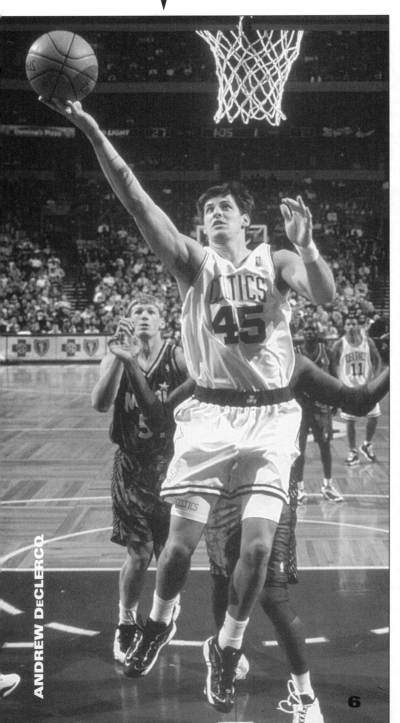

ANDREW DeCLERCQ

Andrew DeClercq, who played a season and a half with the Celtics before being traded to the Cleveland Cavaliers, knows how important it is for him to do whatever he can to avoid injuries. Playing basketball is his livelihood. And if stretching for an extra twenty minutes before the game or practice will help, it's definitely worth it. "Andrew is very cognizant of how important it is to stay healthy," Ed Lacerte, DeClercq's trainer when he was with the Celtics, says. "He knows he had to maximize what he has and he has really put the time and effort into what he is doing. And it has helped his game."

Another player who Lacerte has worked with, Robert Parish, is a prime example of how good body awareness and flexibility due to stretching can prolong a career. Parish played in the NBA for twenty-one years, and, according to Lacerte, was very much in tune with his body."

He could sit on the floor with his legs spread, and touch his chest and stomach to the floor," Lacerte recalls.

Stretching Techniques

We live in an instant gratification society, and perhaps that's why stretching is not as highly valued as it should be. But as Celtics trainer Ed Lacerte says, "If patience is a virtue, then the virtuous will receive the most out of stretching."

Stretching is a discipline that requires you to slow down. It is not an exercise that can be hurried. Indeed, everyone has probably seen people in gyms use a bouncing effect while they stretch, especially when they lean over and try to touch their toes. That is a product of being in a hurry. The process is called ballistic stretching, and it is a good indication that the person has no idea what he or she is doing. Our muscles have a built-in safety feature called the stretch reflex that initiates a contraction in a muscle if it's stretched too quickly. So, anyone who bounces while stretching initiates this response, and instead of stretching a muscle, this method actually causes muscles to contract and become tight. At worst, the ballistic stretch will cause injury before the stretch reflex can counter the movement.

Proper stretching—taking your time—will increase the mobility of your body and will help you to become a better athlete, regardless of your sport. But the slow stretching of muscles is a discipline. It is accomplished by stretching the muscle beyond its resting position, gently but forcibly, to a greater length. It cannot be done too quickly and must be performed on a regular basis with gradual progression to glean the benefits.

ANTAWN JAMISON

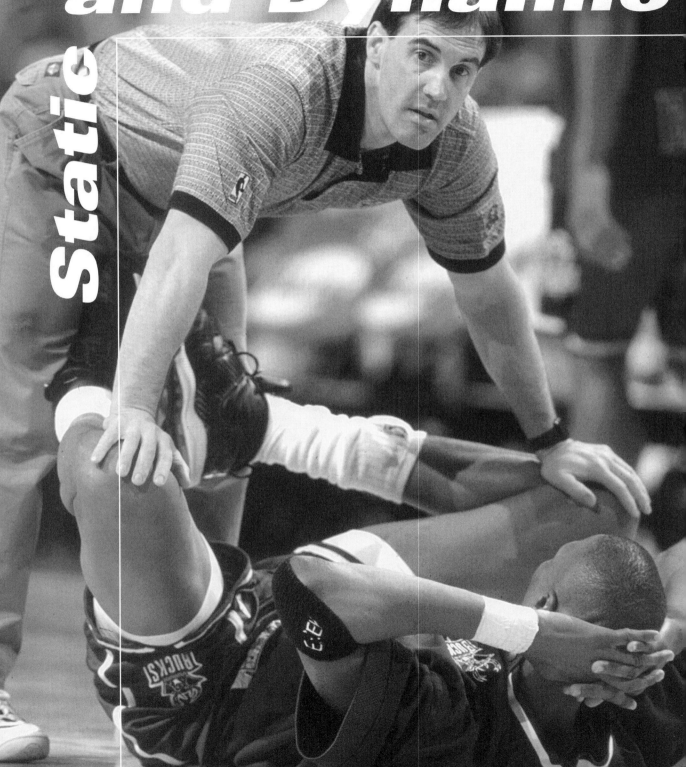

Static **and Dynamic**

Stretching

In technical terms, the two main types of flexibility are called static and dynamic. Static flexibility is the range of motion around a joint or a series of joints, and is limited by the ability of the muscles to stretch. Dynamic flexibility describes the active motion around a joint or series of joints and is limited by, among other things, the resistance to motion of the joint structure.

Static stretching, which should be relaxing and serves the purpose of relieving soreness, holds your muscle in a fixed range of motion for a certain amount of time. One example is lifting the leg and keeping it high without any support. Keep in mind that static stretches will improve your static flexibility, but not necessarily your dynamic flexibility.

Dynamic stretching, which is a more aggressive form, involves stretches that are performed through a wider range of motion. They stimulate the nervous system in the joints, with the goal of increasing range of motion and speed of movement through sport-specific actions. Examples of dynamic stretches are arm swings and leg raises.

If you are working out with a partner, you can utilize a process called passive partner stretching, which is designed to increase your range of motion by having a partner stretch your muscles for you. This is better than stretching by yourself because it is easier for a partner to isolate a particular muscle to stretch.

> Keep in mind that static stretches will improve your static flexibility, but not necessarily your dynamic flexibility.

Warm-Up

Using various dynamic stretches as a warm-up prior to physical activity is recommended, but it's also important to have a brief warm-up even before you start stretching. As we've discussed, warm muscles stretch more easily than cold ones. Connective tissue is like plastic, which when warm is much more pliable. Take a few minutes to jog, bike, jump rope, do calisthenics, or run in place to make the stretching process more productive. All you need is enough time to increase your body temperature, which allows your muscles to work more efficiently.

On the following pages are stretching exercises, listed by the different parts of the body, that will help you prepare for your workout or competition, regardless of your particular sport. A number of the static stretches can be performed as dynamic exercises by continuing the motion instead of holding a stretch.

The Whens and Hows of Stretching.

When to stretch?
- Before and after your game or workout

How often to stretch?
- Every day

How long to stretch?
- 20 seconds for most stretches, 30 for sport-specific stretches

How many repetitions per stretching position?
- Three for longer duration stretches
- Six to twelve for shorter duration stretches

Exercises

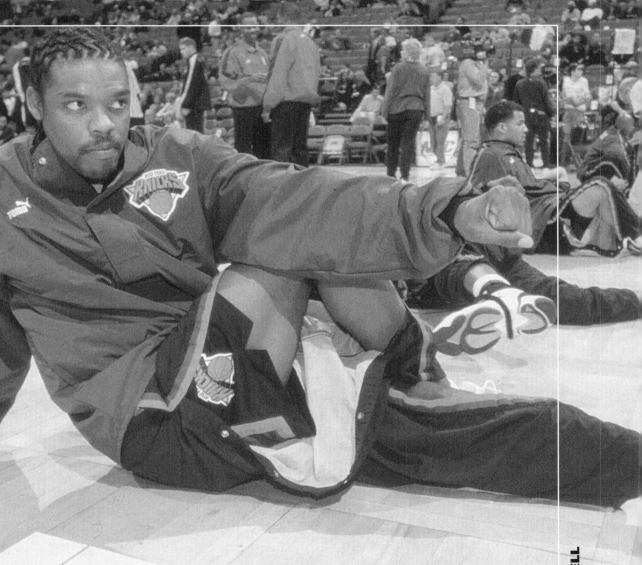

LATRELL SPREWELL

Shoulders

Standing Arm Circles

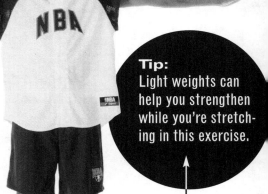

Starting Position: Stand straight up with your feet shoulder-width apart and your arms extended parallel to the floor.

Movement/Stretch: Slowly swing your arms in forward circles, increasing the size of the circles as you exercise. Now reverse the direction.

Tip: Light weights can help you strengthen while you're stretching in this exercise.

Chest

Standing Arm Lifts Behind Back

Starting Position: Standing straight up, place both arms straight behind your back and fold your hands while leaning your upper torso forward.

Movement: Keeping your head upright and your neck relaxed, slowly raise your straight arms behind you as high as you can.

Stretch: Hold the stretch for twenty to thirty seconds.

Tip: Make sure your arms are as straight as you can make them in this exercise. Stop if you're feeling a pinching or irritation in your shoulder.

Trunk/Upper Back

Standing (or Sitting) Arm Across Chest

Starting Position:
Stand or sit up straight with
your hands at your sides.

Movement/Stretch: Lift your right arm and
cross it in front of your upper chest until it is
parallel to the floor. Flex your left arm at the
elbow and grasp your right triceps with your left
hand. Slowly pull your right arm to the left farther
across your chest until you feel the stretch in your
upper back and triceps. Hold the stretch for twenty
to thirty seconds. Repeat with your left arm.

Tip: Your chin should be
approximately on top of
and between your biceps
and shoulder at
the beginning of the
movement.

Standing (or Sitting) Arms Above Head

Starting Position: Stand or sit up straight
with your hands at your sides.

Movement/Stretch: Fold your hands
in front of your torso and slowly turn
and lift them until your arms are at full
extension and your hands are directly
above your head, palms up. Stretch
upward with your hands and arms
and slowly reach slightly backward.
Hold the stretch for twenty to
thirty seconds.

Tip: Keep
your hands folded
during the entire
exercise.

13

Lower Back/Hips/Gluteals

Lying Low Back Stretch

Starting Position: Lie flat on your back on the floor or a mat with your legs extended and together, your toes pointing straight up and your hands at your sides.

Movement/Stretch: Flex your right knee and bring it up toward your chest. Grasp your right knee with folded hands and pull it as close to your chest as you can. Hold the stretch for twenty to thirty seconds. Repeat with the left leg. Then repeat with both legs simultaneously, pulling your right knee back with your right hand and your left knee back with your left hand and lifting your tailbone slightly.

Tip: Keep the back of your head flat on the floor or a mat during all three of these exercises. Hold in your abdominal muscles. For a slight variation, alternate bringing your knee toward the shoulder or armpit instead of the chest.

Lying Crossover

Starting Position: Lie flat on your back on the floor or a mat with your legs extended and together and your toes pointing straight up. Your arms should be straight out to the sides and your palms flat on the floor.

Movement/Stretch: Keeping your legs straight, rotate your right hip and slowly swing your right leg over your left leg so that your right foot comes close to touching your left hand. Keep your upper back, shoulders, and back of your head flat on the floor during this movement. Then move your right foot even closer to your left hand. Hold the stretch for twenty to thirty seconds. Swing your right leg back to its original position. Repeat with your left leg.

Tip: Your non-swinging leg can turn slightly outward during the swing, but try to keep all other areas of your body still to maximize the effect in the buttocks and hip.

Groin/Inner Thigh

Yoga

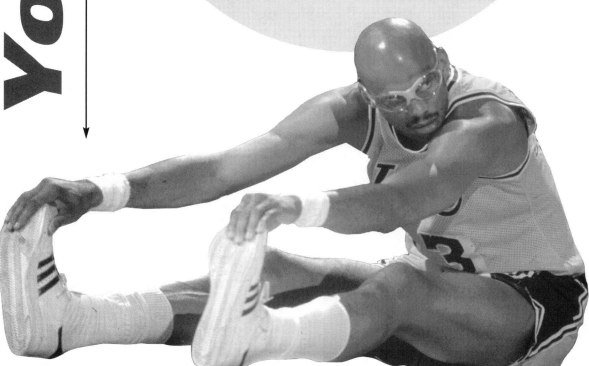

Always ahead of his time, Hall-of-Famer Kareem Abdul-Jabbar, who played twenty years in the NBA and is the all-time leading scorer, credits his playing longevity to his practice of yoga and the martial arts. Abdul-Jabbar also meditated before every game to reduce stress. Yoga, breathing exercises, meditation, martial arts, and other Eastern techniques are just now being discovered by NBA trainers, coaches, and players, and incorporated into training practices.

Groin/Inner Thigh

Sitting Spread-Eagle ◄──────────────────────────┐

Starting Position: Sit up straight on the floor with your legs extended and spread out as far as possible, and your feet pointing up and slightly out.

First Movement/Stretch: Leaning your upper torso toward your right leg with your head pointed directly toward your right foot, reach with both hands and grasp toward your right foot. Hold the stretch for twenty to thirty seconds. Repeat with your left leg.

Second Movement/Stretch: From the same starting position, lean your upper torso forward with your head pointed to a midpoint between your feet and reach as far as you can with your right hand toward your right foot and your left hand toward your left foot. Hold the stretch for twenty to thirty seconds.

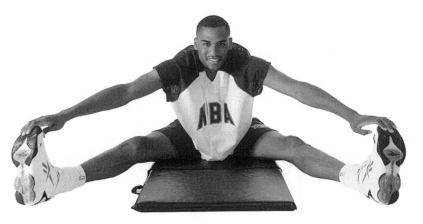

Tip: If you can't reach your toes in these positions, grasp your ankle or calf instead. You'll still get a good groin and inner thigh stretch out of these exercises. If you are able to reach your toes, pull them back gently.

Sitting Butterflies ←

Starting Position: Sit on the floor with your knees bent and to the sides and the bottoms of your feet together. Pull your feet toward your body and place your hands on your ankles, your forearms on your inner calves, and your elbows on your inner knees.

Movement/Stretch: Lean your upper torso forward from the hips to apply pressure with your forearms and elbows to push your knees toward the floor as much as possible. Hold the stretch for twenty to thirty seconds.

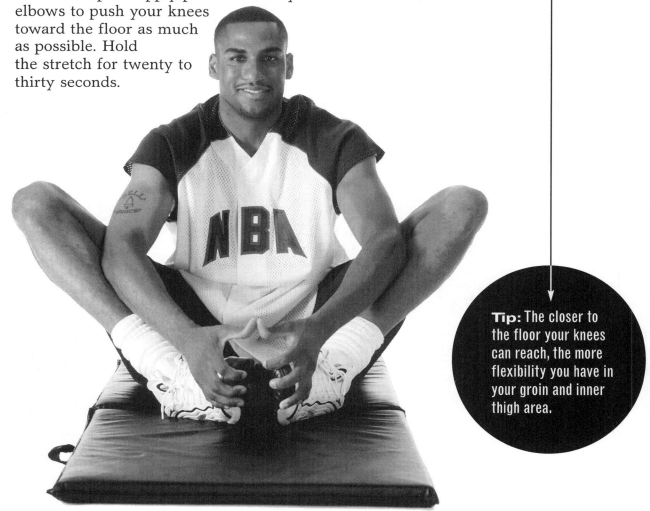

Tip: The closer to the floor your knees can reach, the more flexibility you have in your groin and inner thigh area.

Hamstrings

Sitting Leg-In Stretch ←

Starting Position: Sit up straight on the floor with your left leg tucked in and your right leg extended and your toes pointing up.

First Movement/Stretch: Leaning your upper torso forward from the hips, grasp toward the toes of your right foot with your right hand, while your left hand rests on the floor by your left foot. Pull your chest toward your leg. Hold the stretch for twenty to thirty seconds.

Second Movement/Stretch: From the same starting position, lean your upper torso forward from the hips and grasp your right ankle with both hands, pulling your chest toward your leg. Hold the stretch for twenty to thirty seconds.

Third Movement/Stretch: From the same starting position, lean your upper torso forward from the hips and grasp your right ankle with both hands and pull your chest toward your leg, but this time point your toes away from your body. Hold the stretch for twenty to thirty seconds. Following all three movements, repeat with your left leg.

Tip: If you are able to reach your toes, pull them back gently.

Lying Leg-Up Stretch

Starting Position: Lie flat on your back on the floor or a mat with your knees just slightly bent and your toes pointing up.

First Movement/Stretch: Raise your right leg and bring your knee toward your chest. When your thigh is ninety degrees to your body, slowly extend your leg straight up and grasp it with both hands directly behind your knee. Point your toes up and contract your calf muscle. Hold the stretch for twenty to thirty seconds.

Tip: Pointing your toes up and toward your head will make you feel the stretch in different areas of the hamstring. Don't force the stretch into the pain area.

Second Movement/Stretch: Maintaining the same position, point your toes toward your head. Repeat both movements with your left leg.

Quadriceps

Standing Quad Stretch

Starting Position: Stand straight up and place your right hand against a wall in front of you. The toes of your left foot should be pointing forward toward the wall.

Movement/Stretch: Bending at the knee, raise your right foot back and up and grasp it with your left hand behind you. Slowly pull your right foot toward your left buttocks as far as you can. Hold the stretch for twenty to thirty seconds. Repeat with your left leg and right hand.

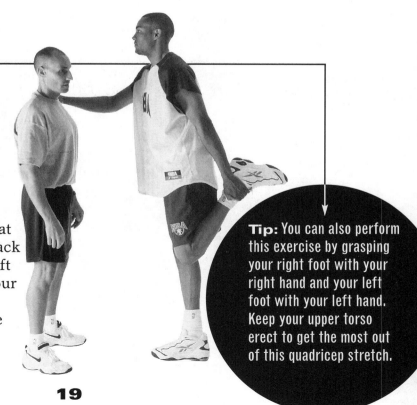

Tip: You can also perform this exercise by grasping your right foot with your right hand and your left foot with your left hand. Keep your upper torso erect to get the most out of this quadricep stretch.

Calf/Lower Leg

Sitting Towel Stretch ←

Starting Position: Sit straight up on the floor with your left leg tucked in and your right leg extended in front of you and your toes pointing up.

Movement/Stretch: Leaning slightly forward, wrap a towel around the ball of your right foot and hold the towel with both hands. Pull back gently on the towel until you feel the stretch in your calf and Achilles tendon area. Hold the stretch for twenty to thirty seconds. Repeat with your left leg.

Tip: Don't yank on the towel, which can cause damage to the Achilles tendon and calf muscles. Don't let the towel slip down to the sole of your foot.

Standing Wall Lean

Starting Position: Standing directly in front of and facing a wall, lean your upper torso forward, put your hands against the wall.

Movement/Stretch: Bend your left knee slightly and slide your right leg as far back as you can while keeping your right foot flat on the floor. Hold the stretch for twenty to thirty seconds. Repeat with your left leg.

Tip: Keep your toes pointed toward the wall and your feet flat on the floor at all times, that is, heels down.

Chapter 2

Aerobic and Cardiovascular

Robert Parish

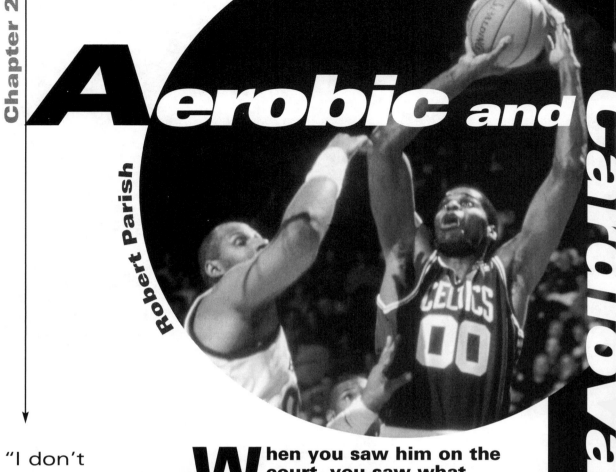

"I don't allow myself to get out of shape."

Robert Parish, who played twenty-one years in the NBA.

When you saw him on the court, you saw what seemed like the perfect human specimen. He was buff. He was toned. He worked hard in the weight room. He ate well and took vitamin supplements. He didn't drink. He didn't smoke. He appeared invincible. Yet every season he would go down with an injury that would take him off the court for long periods of time. He couldn't understand it. He thought he was doing the right thing. That he was treating his body like a temple. Why was he always getting injured? And then you discovered that with all the weight lifting, the supplements, and a proper diet, he was neglecting something that was far more important than anything else. He was neglecting his heart.

"I pride myself on conditioning and working out, being ready to play," says Karl Malone of the Utah Jazz. "I was curious to know what it would be like during the 1998–1999 season with the compact, shortened schedule. My body held up well." Karl Malone says his body fat is 3.6 percent.

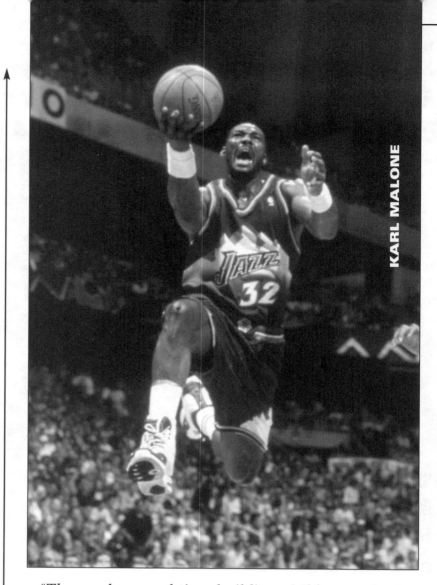

KARL MALONE

"Those who spend time building visible muscles in order to beat their opponents in games often ignore the invisible muscle that beats to give them vitality in life," says Chris Tucker, head athletic trainer for the Atlanta Hawks. Blown-out knees, strains and sprains, shortness of breath, and even heart attacks are not uncommon problems for athletes who may know enough to stretch, strengthen some muscles, eat right and wear protective equipment, but don't understand the importance of shaping up their most important muscle with consistent aerobic activity.

The primary reason for injuries is fatigue, and fatigue comes from a heart out of shape. Shin splints usually occur near the end of the race; football and basketball injuries frequently happen in the fourth quarter; and skiers often get hurt at the bottom of the hill. It takes cardiovascular fitness to reduce fatigue, which in turn will reduce injuries.

Aerobics

What is aerobics? It's the promotion of the supply of oxygen-rich blood from the heart to the muscles. The more of this oxygen-rich blood that can be supplied, the more efficiently the body can use it, leading to cardiovascular or cardiorespiratory fitness. *Aerobics* means "working with oxygen," while *cardio* refers to the heart, *vascular* to the blood vessels, and *respiratory* to the lungs.

Aerobics not only increases the heart's ability to pump blood, it also makes muscle tissues more efficient at oxidizing body fat. A large, healthy heart can pump large volumes of oxygen-rich blood with each beat. Aerobic exercise raises the body's level of high-density lipoproteins ("good cholesterol") and reduces triglyceride levels, while at the same time raising testosterone levels to help muscles store energy in the form of glycogen.

Aerobic conditioning employed at sixty to eighty percent of maximum heart rate capacity for fifteen or more minutes per day several times a week will strengthen the cardiovascular system significantly and make us healthier and better athletes.

> "In the summertime, I do not shoot basketballs. It's all conditioning."
>
> *Moses Malone, nineteen-year veteran and eleven-time NBA All-Star.*

Off-Season Workouts

"One of the most fitness-conscious guys on the Hawks is Dikembe Mutombo," says Chris Tucker. "He works out every day [during the off-season] and even manages a routine on game days during the season.

Doug Christie, a seven-year veteran who plays for the Toronto Raptors, is also a huge proponent of off-season conditioning. "Off-season conditioning prevents injuries and helps you withstand the grueling demands of a season," said Christie. "It also puts you into a confident frame of mind. If you're in shape, you feel good, and it's easier to give your best on the court."

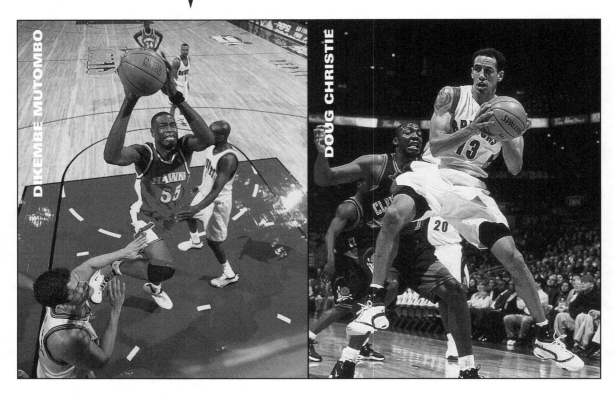

DIKEMBE MUTOMBO

DOUG CHRISTIE

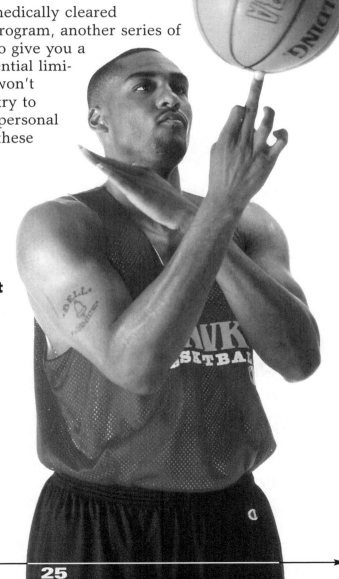

The first step before you begin a cardiovascular regimen is to see your doctor for a physical so he can rule out any possible medical problems that might result from beginning or stepping up your exercise program. Virtually everyone will see his health and performance improve with an aerobic program, but a small minority could be predisposed to heart problems with the onset of an increased workload.

Once you've been medically cleared to initiate an exercise program, another series of tests is recommended to give you a better idea of your potential limitations. If your doctor won't administer these tests, try to enlist the services of a personal fitness trainer. Among these measurements are:

- **Body fat**

- **Flexibility**

- **Strength tests**

- **Girth measurement**

- **Conditioning**

- **Walk test**

- **Run test**

- **Heart rate maintenance**

Heart Rate

By improving your entire cardiovascular system with aerobic training, you can make your heart a more efficient machine. As your heart rate goes down, your overall condition improves. Lowering your resting heart rate through exercise allows for a longer rest interval between heart beats, giving the heart chambers more time to fill with your blood before it's pumped out. This results in a greater ejection of oxygen-rich blood to your lungs and the rest of your body.

In order to maximize your aerobic workout, it's important to stay within a certain heart rate range for at least fifteen minutes. Most of the experts recommend exercising at sixty to eighty percent of your maximal heart rate.

To determine your heart rate during and after exercise, you can take your pulse. Immediately after exercising, take your pulse for fifteen seconds and multiply it by four. If you are an advanced athlete, take it for six seconds and multiply it by ten. The best place to find your pulse is at the carotid artery in the neck. That method, however, can be unreliable. The most effective and reliable way to measure heart rate is with a heart rate monitor.

Heart Rate Monitors

There are two types of heart rate monitors: the electrode chest belt and the photocell. The photocell monitor utilizes a photocell sensor and a light source placed on the earlobe or finger to measure heart rate. The electrode chest belt utilizes two electrodes mounted on a sealed electrode transmitter attached to the chest with an elastic belt. These electrodes pick up electrical impulses from the heart and relay the information via an electromagnetic field to a wrist monitor.

"For my Atlanta Hawks players, heart rate monitoring turned the drudgery of the treadmill into a fun competition," Chris Tucker says.

Using a heart rate monitor will allow you to understand your body's capabilities and to measure the improvement your cardiorespiratory system is making over time.

"For my Atlanta Hawks players, heart rate monitoring turned the drudgery of the treadmill into a fun competition," Chris Tucker says. "Even though basketball players will run all day while they're playing, put them on a treadmill and they get bored very quickly. But when we put all of them on the machines and we tell them that no one's heart rate can drop below 160 for a designated period of time, suddenly they're focused because it's a challenge and a competition."

Coach Pat Riley is a big proponent of fitness training, and Tim Hardaway has blossomed under him.

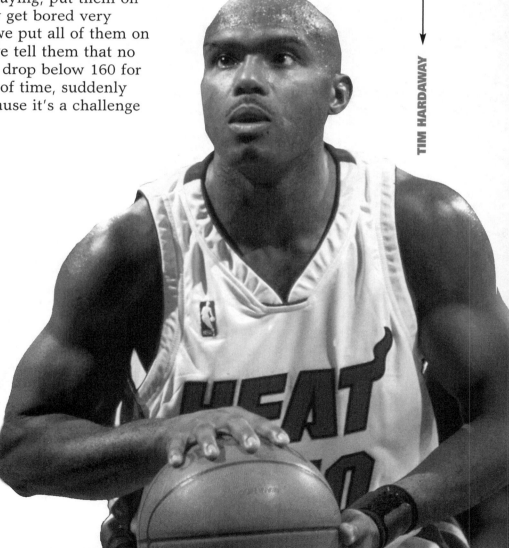

TIM HARDAWAY

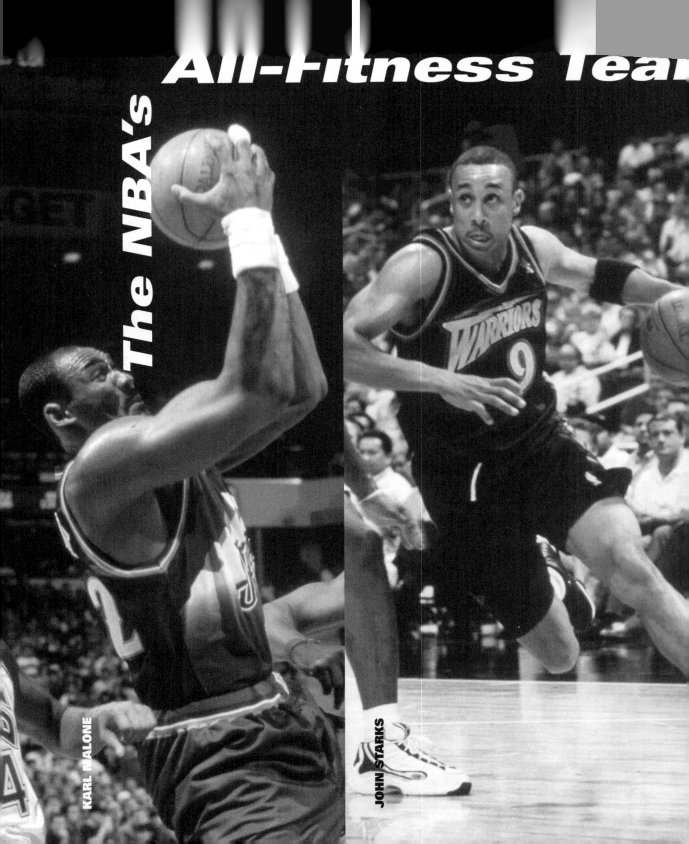

KARL MALONE

JOHN STARKS

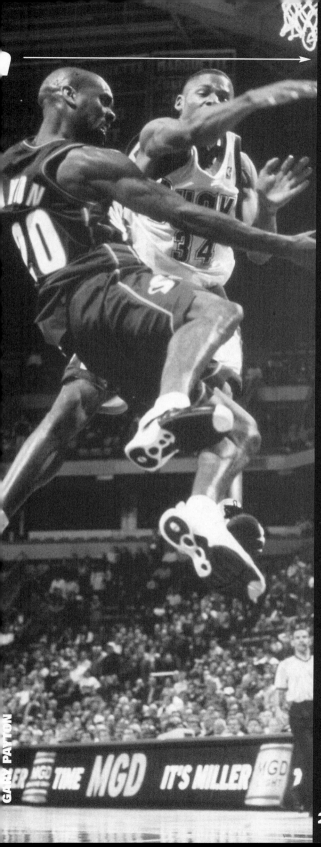

Karl Malone—I use him as an example of how a big man should train.

Mookie Blaylock—He's one of the hardest workers I've been around and he likes to train alone.

Alonzo Mourning—All the Georgetown guys, Mourning, Ewing, and Mutombo are hard workers, but Zo probably works the hardest.

Gary Payton—He's a flash on the court, and that comes with hard work.

Tyrone Corbin—He works out every day, and after fourteen years in the league has never had a major injury.

Chris Mullin—I've seen a couple of his workouts; they're very intense. If he didn't work so hard, he probably wouldn't have come back from so many injuries.

Tim Hardaway—Pat Riley is a big proponent of fitness training, and Hardaway has blossomed under him.

John Starks—A hard worker, and it shows with his effort on the court.

Steve Smith—Making the All-Star team with his bad knees is a testament to how hard he worked.

Michael Jordan—Even in retirement, he's still one of the fittest in the league.

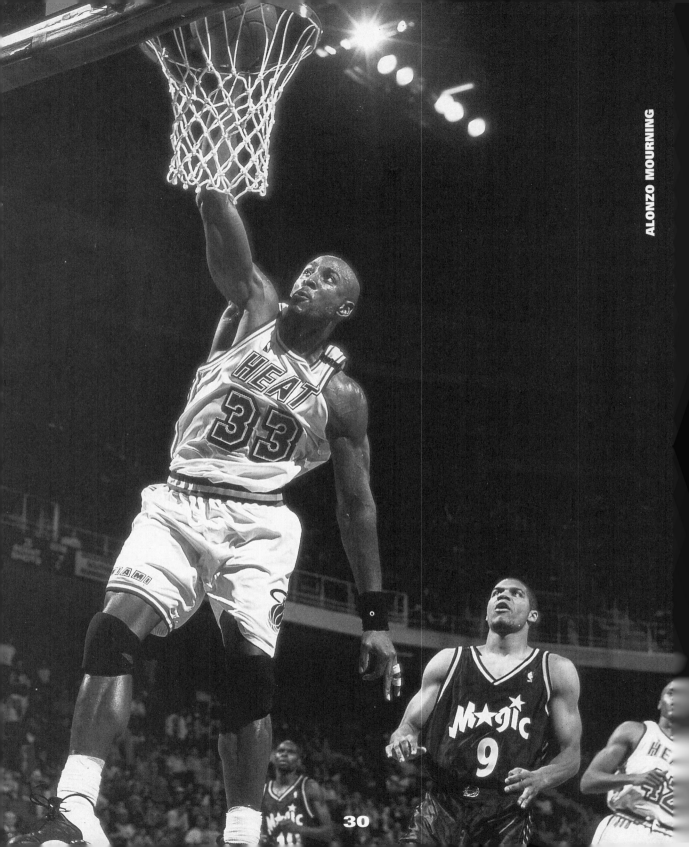

ALONZO MOURNING

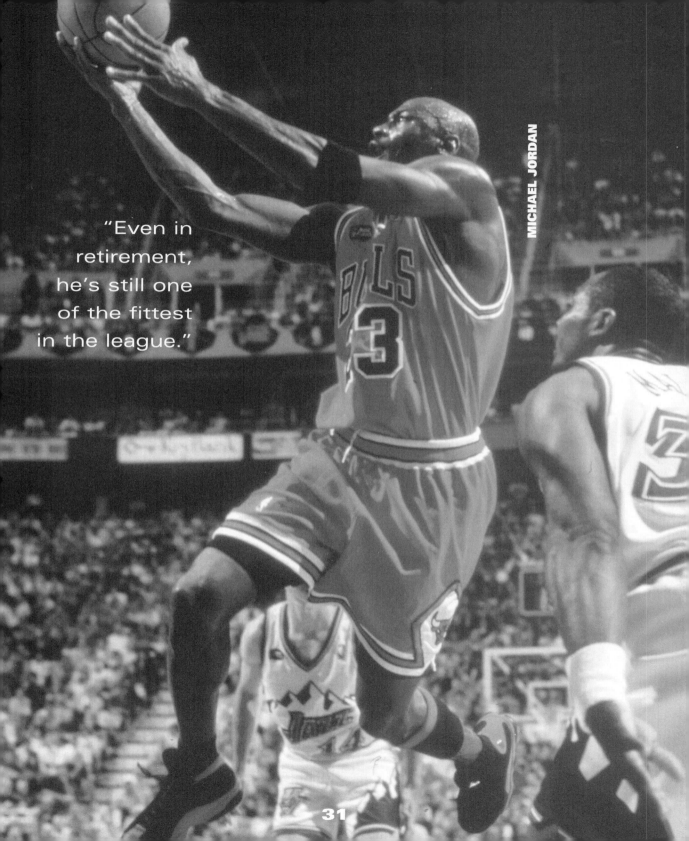

"Even in retirement, he's still one of the fittest in the league."

MICHAEL JORDAN

31

Now that you've been cleared by a doctor for aerobic exercise, you understand the importance of getting into shape aerobically and decided upon a program that will get you there in a few short months. You're ready to walk or jog; or run; or hit the bike or treadmill or pool, right? Wait a minute. Actually, wait five minutes because that is what is recommended for a very important pre-exercise warm-up each time you work out or compete.

The purpose of the warm-up is literally to "warm" your body, including both your general body temperature and your deep muscle-tissue temperature. This will prepare your body for the somewhat more strenuous activity to come. A warm-up will increase your metabolism, oxygen uptake, blood flow, nerve impulses, motor units of muscle fiber, adrenaline, and blood sugar.

In this warm-up, you want to stretch your muscles and get your heart rate up slightly. For a complete stretching routine, see Chapter 1.

If you are just beginning to get serious about aerobic training, begin at sixty percent of your maximum heart rate and exercise for fifteen minutes per day for two days a week, preferably with several days in between workouts. Maximum heart rate can be determined by subtracting your age from 220. The fat-burning areas occur in the sixty to seventy percent range. Do this for two weeks and then you'll be ready to increase the intensity of your program.

HAKEEM OLAJUWON

Walking

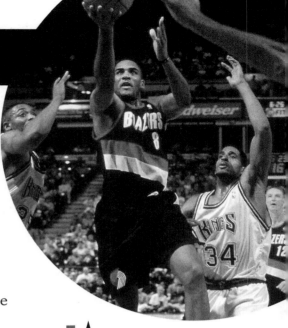

Steve Smith of the Portland Trail Blazers has had numerous knee injuries. As part of his conditioning regimen, running was his primary activity. Now, however, he has become a converted walker. And walking, according to Smith's trainer when he was with the Hawks, Chris Tucker, is one of the best aerobic exercises you can do. "I'm a big fan of walking," Tucker says. "With walking you can go longer than with running, and it takes much less of a toll on the body than running does. You'll work every muscle in your legs by walking, as well as abdominals and back muscles, which are working to keep your body upright. A half hour of vigorous walking can burn between 180 and 250 calories."

And Steve Smith, even with those damaged knees, was an All-Star in 1998 and is a member of the 2000 U.S. Men's National Team.

After two weeks of fifteen minutes of aerobic exercise per day twice a week, you'll be ready to move on. At this point either add five minutes to your workout or add a third day to the week. After two more weeks you can add whichever element you didn't add last time, so you should now be exercising for twenty minutes per session three days a week.

If you're a more serious athlete who's already pretty well fit aerobically, start with thirty minutes a day three times a week and build from there. Either way, the goal is to get to five days a week (all in a row) with 45 to 60 consecutive minutes of aerobic exercise per session. It will probably take you several months to reach this stage, but when you do, you'll already be feeling healthier and will probably see improved performance in your individual sport.

STEVE SMITH

Tucker says, "With walking you can go longer than with running, and it takes much less of a toll on the body than running does."

Chris Tucker's Eight Principles of Aerobic Exercises

- **Intensity:**
  How hard are you working?

- **Frequency:**
  How often do you work out?

- **Duration:**
  How many minutes per workout?

- **Variation:**
  Vary your workout routine.

- **Specificity:**
  Find the workout that best mimics your sport.

- **Progression:**
  Keep making progress.

- **Overload:**
  Always try to do a little more than you did last time.

- **Individuality:**
  Don't worry what others are doing; do what's best for you.

CHRIS MULLIN

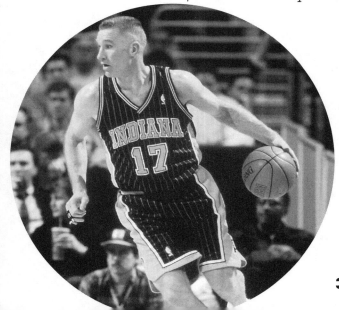

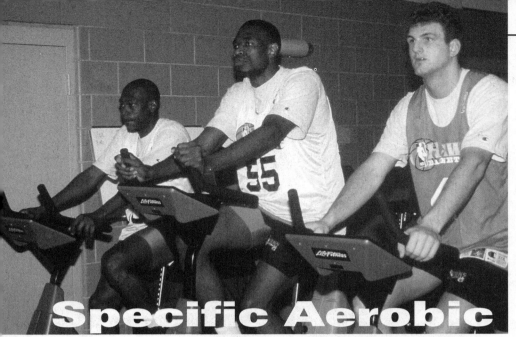

Specific Aerobic Exercises

Hopping around a gymnasium in tights like a character in Peter Pan just might not appeal to you. It doesn't have to. You can become aerobically fit without ever performing aerobic exercises you've seen late at night on infomercials. You can achieve the cardiovascular fitness that will transform you into a better athlete by exercising in a variety of ways. You can walk, hike, jog, run, cycle, row, ski, swim, or use equipment such as the treadmill, stair climber, stationary bike, or rowing machine. And you can use any number of these exercises in combination with each other.

"I'm a big proponent of variation during a workout," says Chris Tucker. "With the Hawks, our workouts are never the same. One day we might bike for fifteen minutes, do the treadmill for fifteen, then go to the track and do some other things. Or we'll bike for 25 minutes, then do some sprint work, then hit the weights. And it doesn't matter if you're an NBA player or Joe weekend athlete; you need to get going. And you've got to change your workout because I don't care who you are, you're going to get bored and quit if you don't."

You can walk, hike, jog, run, cycle, row, ski, swim, or use equipment such as the treadmill, stair climber, stationary bike, or rowing machine.

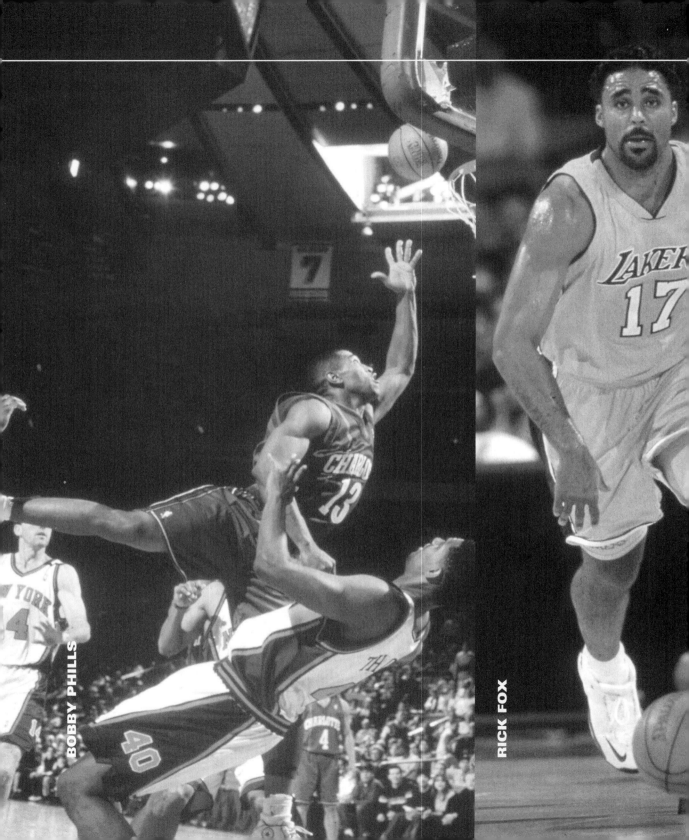

BOBBY PHILLS

RICK FOX

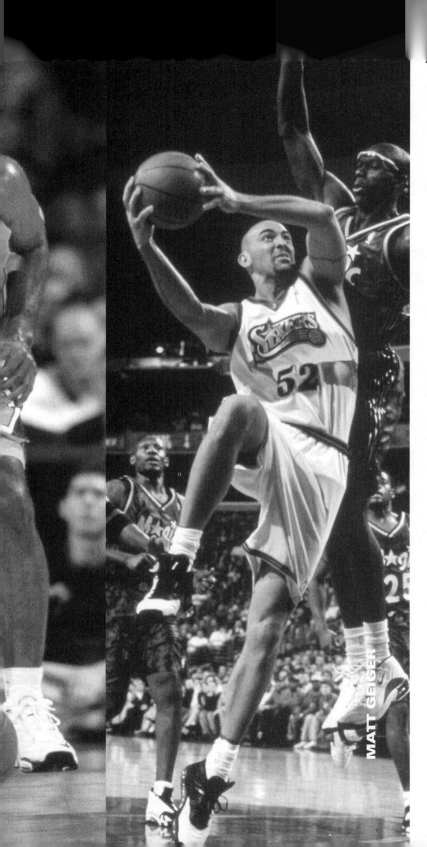

MATT GEIGER

As Chris Tucker said, keeping your workout the same can be tedious and possibly counterproductive. There are other ways to work your body that can be more enjoyable as well as beneficial. Here is a sampling of players and some of their favorite physical activities aside from basketball.

Bobby Phills, Charlotte Hornets: swimming

Christian Laettner, Detroit Pistons: snow-boarding

Jud Buechler, Detroit Pistons: volleyball

Matt Geiger, Philadelphia 76ers: hydrosliding

Dirk Nowitzki, Dallas Mavericks: European hand-ball

Rick Fox, Los Angeles Lakers: martial arts

Bimbo Coles, Atlanta Hawks: baseball

Malik Rose, San Antonio Spurs: playing the tuba, sax, and trombone (good work-out for the mouth, lungs, and arms)

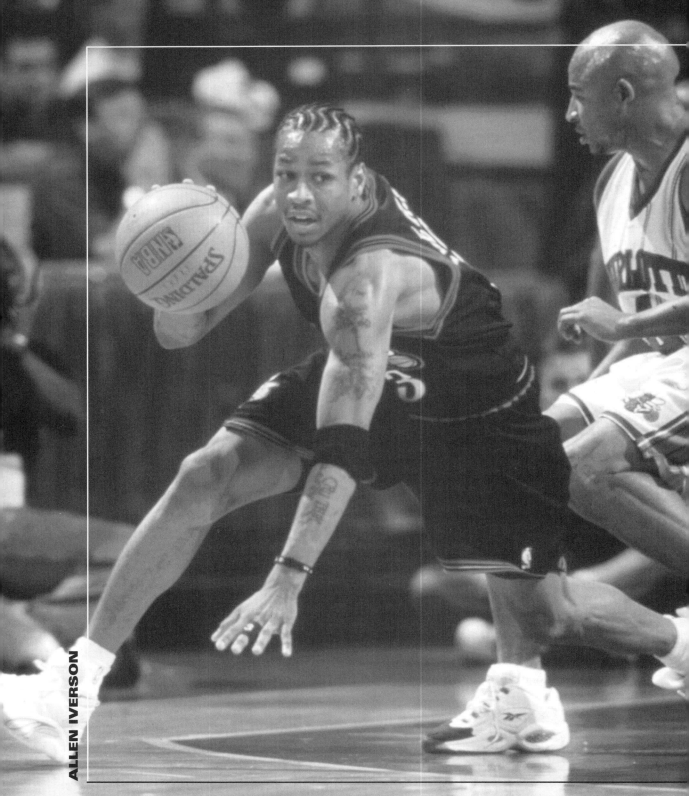

ALLEN IVERSON

Order of Exercises

Once you've determined the various muscles you're going to exercise during an aerobic workout, decide on an order that makes sense. It's best to work the large muscle groups first, then the smaller ones. If you work your calves before you work your hips and quads, or if you concentrate on your biceps and triceps before your back, you may be too fatigued to work the larger muscles you should.

SHAQUILLE O'NEAL

Chris Tucker's Aerobic Fitness

The following are aerobic exercises suggested by Chris Tucker, and from which you can select to form your own personal training circuits that you can do at the gym or at home if you have the necessary equipment.

These exercises are divided among beginner, intermediate, and advanced. If you're a beginner, your goal should be to achieve improved cardiovascular fitness in approximately six months. Use the first two months to perform beginner circuits (15–30 minutes), the third and fourth months to perform intermediate circuits (30–45 minutes), and the fifth and sixth months to perform advanced circuits (45 minutes to an hour).

When putting together your training circuits, try to alternate the strength exercises (sit-ups, push-ups, weights, etc.) with your more traditional aerobic exercises (treadmill, bike, StairMaster, etc.), and also alternate between machines and free weights, as well as on-floor and off-floor exercises. You might want to concentrate on your upper body one day and your lower body the next, rather than going for a full-body workout every time. Even if you do not have access to any machines, bikes, or weights, you can always get a good cardiovascular workout by just jogging. *Doing* the workout is more important than *how* you do it.

Training Circuits

Beginner Aerobic Exercises

Treadmill walk (3 minutes)

Sit-ups (25 repetitions)

Stationary bike (3 minutes)

Push-ups (10 reps)

Jump rope or Mini-trampoline jog (2 minutes)

Quadricep extensions (10 reps)

Hamstring curls (10 reps)

Front lat pull-down or One-arm dumbbell row (10 reps)

StairMaster or Run in place with high knees (3 minutes)

Squat (10 reps)*

Rowing (3 minutes)

Front lunge (10 reps)

Alternated dumbbell curl (10 reps)**

Stationary bike or Versa Climber (3 minutes)

Barbell toe raise (10 reps) ***

Step-ups with barbell (10 reps)****

Alternated dumbbell press (10 reps)

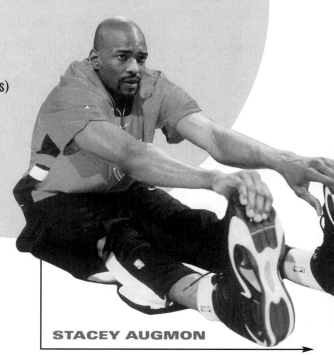

STACEY AUGMON

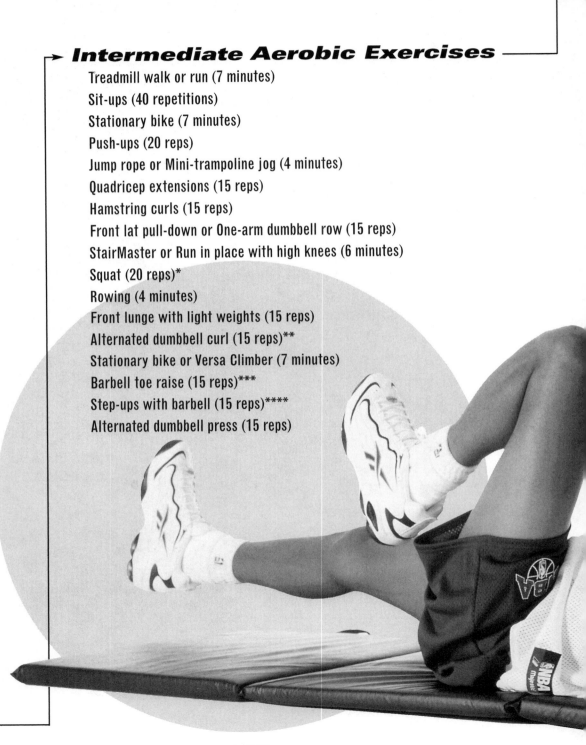

Intermediate Aerobic Exercises

Treadmill walk or run (7 minutes)

Sit-ups (40 repetitions)

Stationary bike (7 minutes)

Push-ups (20 reps)

Jump rope or Mini-trampoline jog (4 minutes)

Quadricep extensions (15 reps)

Hamstring curls (15 reps)

Front lat pull-down or One-arm dumbbell row (15 reps)

StairMaster or Run in place with high knees (6 minutes)

Squat (20 reps)*

Rowing (4 minutes)

Front lunge with light weights (15 reps)

Alternated dumbbell curl (15 reps)**

Stationary bike or Versa Climber (7 minutes)

Barbell toe raise (15 reps)***

Step-ups with barbell (15 reps)****

Alternated dumbbell press (15 reps)

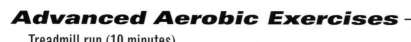

Advanced Aerobic Exercises

Treadmill run (10 minutes)

Sit-ups (50 repetitions)

Stationary bike (10 minutes)

Push-ups (25 reps)

Jump rope or Mini-trampoline jog (5–8 minutes)

Quadricep extensions (20 reps)

Hamstring curls (20 reps)

Front lat pull-down or One-arm dumbbell row (20 reps)

StairMaster or Run in place with high knees (8–10 minutes)

Squat (25 reps)*

Rowing (5 minutes)

Front lunge with light weights (20 reps)

Alternated dumbbell curl (20 reps)**

Stationary bike or Versa Climber (10 minutes)

Barbell toe raise (20 reps)***

Step-ups with barbell (20 reps)****

Alternated dumbbell press (20 reps)

* Can also be performed while holding dumbbells at your sides or a barbell at the back of your neck.

** Can also be performed with barbell, a cable hooked to weights, or on a machine.

*** Can also be performed without a weight, holding dumbbells, or on a stair.

**** Can also be performed without a weight or holding dumbbells.

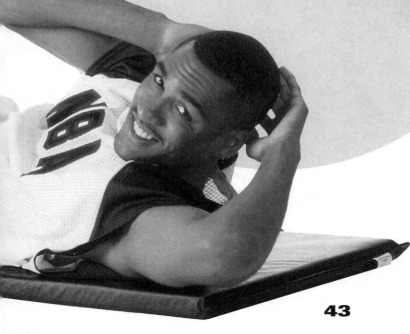

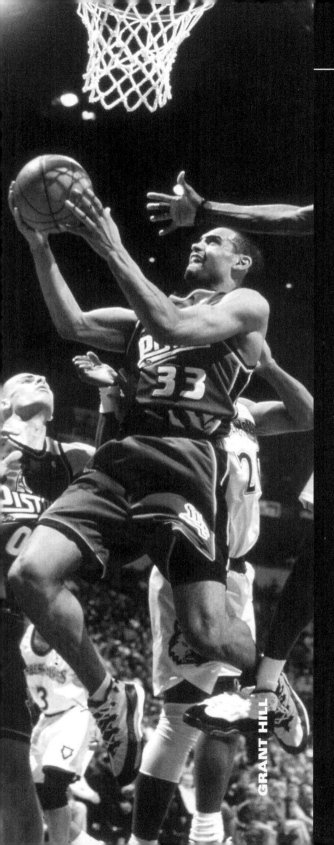

GRANT HILL

The Hoops Workout

Any kind of aerobic workout lasting 15–60 minutes is good for a basketball player, but the aerobic training circuit exercises Chris Tucker recommends for someone whose main sport is hoops would be:

1) On-court running

2) Treadmill

3) Stationary bike

4) StairMaster

5) Pool

Tucker also suggests doing an aerobic conditioning workout on the court. This fifteen-minute, continuous-activity drill would consist of:

1. Run nearly the length of the court and take a shot.

2. Run backward nearly the length of the court and take a shot.

3. Do a defensive slide to the other end of the court and rebound a missed shot.

4. Dribble the length of the court, cutting left and right, then take a shot.

5. Run the length of the court and jump up and touch the backboard three times.

6. Pick up a number of loose balls rolled to you at various areas of the court.

Cool-Down

Some athletes are very consistent with their warm-ups and aerobic fitness routines, but they ignore the important cool-down. The purpose of the cool-down, or recovery period, is to restore your cardiovascular system to near-rest conditions. After working to get the heart to pump blood to the lungs and other areas of the body, it's now time to return blood from the arms and legs to the lungs and heart. There's no better time to stretch your muscles than when they're warm.

"Sometimes it's a battle to get our players to do it," says Chris Tucker of cooling down after a workout. "But some of them love it, including Christian Laettner [now with the Detroit Pistons], who actually looks forward to stretching after a workout. He'll go into a cool, dark room and stretch out all of the muscles he used."

"Training is not something you can overlook. Sometimes it's what keeps you going. Knowing you are improving yourself and your team can be the motivation."

Chris Dudley,
New York Knicks

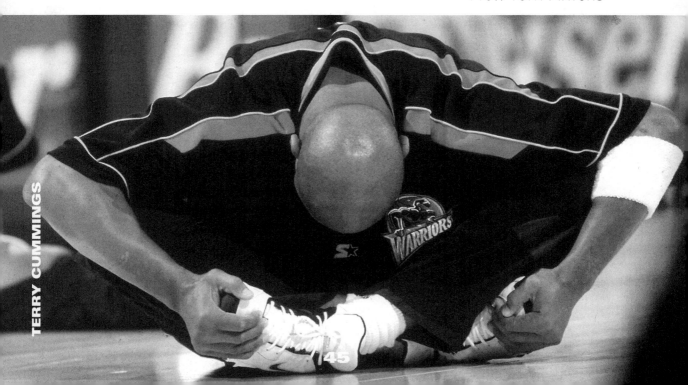

TERRY CUMMINGS

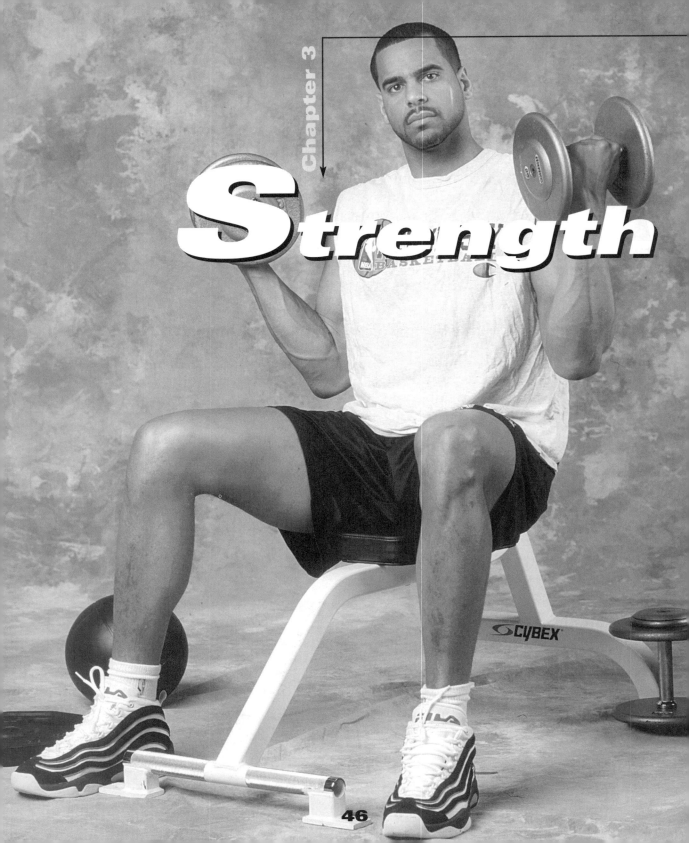

Strength

Training and Weights

The player was a superstar in college. But he played for a very small school in a conference not known for basketball superstars. He was taller and bigger than most of his opposition and he dominated his league. He set records in rebounding and scoring and, despite his small-school background, he was considered a sure thing and was selected in the first round of the NBA draft. When he came to the NBA, however, he struggled. He was consistently out-rebounded by players his size or even smaller, and he had trouble scoring; he just couldn't finish his shots. He was considered a disappointment. Some were even saying he was a flop.

But the following season that same player looked like a new man on the court. He was no longer out-rebounded. His scoring average almost doubled. He had become a very formidable presence on the court. The guy was now a player.

What happened? Why the incredible turnaround?

It seems, coming from that small school in that tiny conference, the player dominated on his size and raw ability. The school had limited sports facilities

JAYSON WILLIAMS

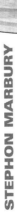

and even less training sophistication. During the off-season after his disastrous rookie year, he worked with his team's trainer on a weight lifting program. He added bulk and strength to his rangy frame, and the results, in his case, were nothing short of miraculous.

Rich Dalatri, assistant coach and strength and training coordinator of the New Jersey Nets, has been in the NBA for twelve years, and he can tell many stories like the one above. He knows, firsthand, how important strength training is in player development.

Take the story of Stephon Marbury, the Nets guard, for example.

"He came out of college after his sophomore year," says Dalatri. "He was a young, scrawny kid. He had no idea what the NBA rigors were going to be like. His game is penetration, dishing to other people, and he was getting killed—really taking a beating. But after that year he went home and got himself into a weight lifting program. The difference now is just incredible: his overall body development, his leg strength, his upper body strength have all improved. When he takes the ball down the lane now, that ball is in a vise. There is nobody in the NBA who comes down the lane as strong as him. He's like a big man. He probably increased his weight from 150-something to around 190. And he did it the correct way. He did it without losing speed, flexibility, or quickness."

Another player Dalatri worked with to help develop his physical strength was Keith Van Horn. "Keith, in his rookie year, did not have a lot of physical, overpowering strength. They were knocking him all over the place," Dalatri recalls. "After that rookie year, we got him on an explosive strength program. Basketball, like most sports, involves considerable movement in the hips, legs, and lower body. If you have a strong base, that will carry you a long way. Keith put a lot of time into hip and leg development. And in his second season he became much more of a presence under the boards."

Perhaps the best example of what strength training can do for an athlete is Michael Jordan and the Chicago Bulls. Michael had a gym built in his home complete with state-of-the-art weight lifting equipment. Not only did Michael use the gym, he insisted that his teammates use it as well. "Some would meet at Michael's house every morning. You just did not get away with not working out," says Dalatri. And the result of all that hard work: six NBA championships.

Though weight lifting and strength training are important, Dalatri stresses that they must work in conjunction with other aspects of a total fitness program. "If you are strong in whatever you do, you are going to be better at what you do," Dalatri says. "But you can be strong and not be flexible; your range of motion will be limited. You can be strong and not have the cardiovascular capacity; if you can't run, you can't play. Or, you can be flexible, have unlimited endurance, but not have the proper strength in your muscles, which will leave you injury prone. Everything must be done together. You can't have one without the other to achieve total fitness."

The purpose of strength training is to produce a natural increase in one's body strength in all of the muscle groups used in your specific sport or sports. Strength training not only increases muscle size, it also strengthens connective tissue and gives joints increased range of motion. The more something is used, the stronger it will get. This is especially true of muscles. And as you become stronger, there is an increase in other areas of fitness as well, including body awareness, balance, speed, and agility. All of the factors you use during compe-

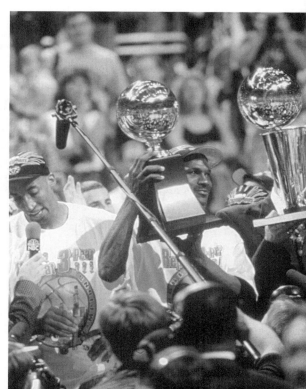

MICHAEL JORDAN AND BULLS WITH TROPHIES

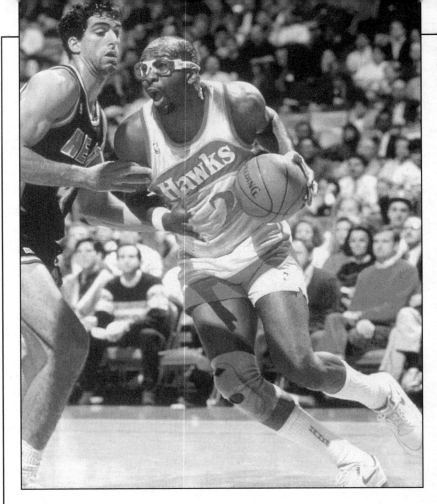

"I think by lifting weights, you get power," says Moses Malone, who played nineteen years in the NBA. "I also think that by lifting, you get focus, direction, discipline, and patience. You get an attitude when you lift weights. You can take the smallest guy in the gym, and if he's lifting weights a lot, he thinks he's bigger."

tition will increase and you'll become a better athlete.

And strength is not only important for competition, but also for overall life fitness. Each part of your body has to have strength to maintain the rigors of everyday life, including your daily routines. Think of all the times you sit in a chair . . . that's squatting. Or lifting those heavy bags of groceries. Or climbing those steps to your apartment. Increased strength will help in ways you probably never even thought of.

the Right Way

Of course, like anything else, strength training needs to be done correctly. If it is, it can go a long way toward helping prevent injuries. If not, it can actually cause injuries. The three biggest problems people have with strength training exercises are:

- Increasing weight too soon
- Doing the repetitions too quickly and not under control
- Doing the exercises incorrectly

Those who attempt exercises too soon or too quickly are usually overanxious, hoping to reach the next level of physical conditioning before they've accomplished the real work necessary to get there. So, they try to perform strength training exercises before they are capable of doing them, or they increase the weight or resistance too rapidly. Others may be ready to take on a particular exercise at a certain level of intensity, but due to improper training or no training at all, they attempt the exercise incorrectly and wind up doing more harm than good.

Getting Started

Prior to doing strength training exercises, it's always a good idea to have a low level, aerobic warm-up of five to ten minutes. Ride a bike, jump rope, jog, walk briskly, or do anything that can get your heart level up and warm your muscles. For more information, see Chapter 2.

CHARLES BARKLEY

The Total Ab Workout

After your aerobic warm-up, you can begin your strength training regimen with abdominal exercises. Ab development is very important. The abs are a muscle group like any other. Exercises that strengthen the abs are ideal as a prelude to weight lifting because they can protect the body from low back injury and help produce stability in the midsection. The following ab circuit will work the lower, middle and upper abs, and obliques (sides).

Abdominal Circuit

1. *Bent Knee Leg Lift.* Lie on floor with hands, palms down, under rear end. Bend knees with feet flat on floor. Raise knees upward to ceiling, keeping the knees at the same angle throughout the movement. Return feet to floor by lowering legs slowly.

2. *Bicycle.* Lie on floor with legs extended flat on the floor. Clasp hands behind head. Raise right shoulder and elbow and move on a diagonal toward left knee, which should, in turn, move toward the right shoulder and elbow. Continue by alternating opposite elbows and knees.

3. *Suitcase.* Lie on floor with knees bent and feet flat on floor, hands clasped behind head. Bring shoulders and chest up while at the same time pulling both knees together. The two parts of the body meet in the middle and the body is in the up position in a V shape. Return to start position slowly.

4. *Leg Up Crunch.* Lie on floor with knees bent, legs lifted off the ground, and hands behind head. Slowly raise your head, shoulders, and upper back off floor by using the abdominal muscles. Hold at top a moment and lower to starting position slowly.

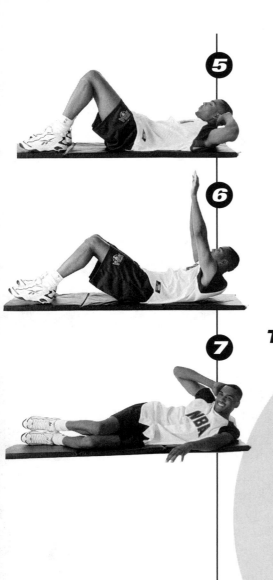

5. *Crunch.* Same as Leg Up Crunch, but with feet flat on the floor.

6. *Reach for Sky.* Lie flat on floor with knees slightly bent and feet flat on floor. Extend arms toward ceiling. Reach upward, raising the shoulders and upper back off the floor. Slowly return to start position.

7. *Side Sit-Ups.* Lie on right side, extend the legs and raise them off the floor approximately six inches. Place left hand behind head. Raise upward to the left and hold for a moment, keeping the legs up at all times. Return slowly to start. Repeat for right side using same procedure.

Those Washboard Abs

Despite what you see on the covers of fitness magazines, or on infomercials on television, those six-pack abs everyone seems to want don't come from sit-ups alone. The best way to tighten your gut and lose flab around the middle is to work hard on burning fat; that translates to more cardiovascular workouts . . . and, of course, eating less fatty foods. But because we know pictures of those ridiculously rippled abs sell, we decided we must include one here. So . . . for your viewing pleasure.

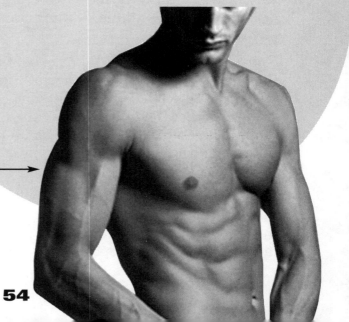

The following is a set of exercises that can be done with either barbells, dumbbells, or the appropriate machines. The exercises recommended here are, according to Rich Dalatri, good to incorporate into an overall fitness program. There are various ways to weight train. Higher weights and lower repetition, one to six reps, will increase size and strength. Moderate repetition, six to twelve reps, will be more beneficial for overall body development and muscle building, while lighter weights and high repetition, above twelve reps, will be more of a cardiovascular workout and help in muscle endurance.

For this workout, Dalatri suggests six to twelve repetitions per set. Beginners should try one to three sets for each exercise; novices, three to four sets; advanced, three to five; with no more than a minute to ninety seconds' rest between each set.

"Start with ridiculously light weights," says Dalatri. "You can always move up. If you go too heavy, you'll get injured or frustrated, which can lead to failure. Know what your level is. Start at a low level. It's like building a pyramid. You have to build the base before the peak."

RICH DALATRI

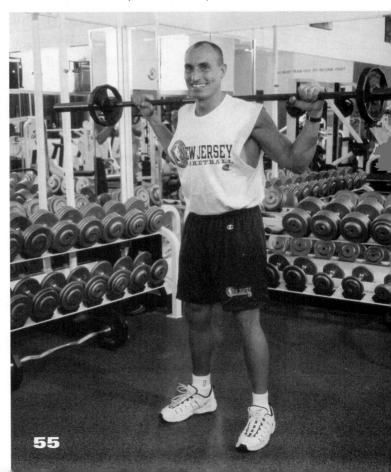

Upper Body

Bench Press (Chest)

Lie on a bench with your feet flat on the floor, grip the bar with a slightly wider than shoulder-width grip. (This grip will give you a good combination of incorporating chest, triceps, lat, and shoulder muscles. A wider grip will concentrate more on the lat and chest muscles. A closer grip will work the shoulders and triceps more.)

Start the exercise by lifting the bar up off the rack and slowly, under control, lowering it to your chest. Touch the bar at mid-chest level. (Do not bounce the weight on your chest.) Pause the bar on your chest a moment, never relaxing or letting the bar crush your chest.

Push the bar upward explosively in a straight line until the last one-third of the extension, when the bar will move slightly toward the rack. (Keep your rear and back in contact with the bench at all times. Feet stay secure on the floor without moving, to ensure a solid base.) Fully extend the arms and pause at the top of the movement before beginning the next repetition.

Incline Press (Chest and Shoulders)

Performed the same as the bench press but on an incline bench. The incline works the muscles of the upper chest and shoulders more than the bench press.

Use a slightly wider than shoulder-width grip. Lift the weights and lower them to the upper portion of your chest. Look at a point on the ceiling and move the bar explosively upward in a straight line to that point. This will ensure you are pushing the weights in a correct angle according to the angle of the bench.

(Be sure to keep your feet secure on the ground and your rear end and back in contact with the bench.)

Military Press (Shoulders)

Grip the bar with a slightly wider than shoulder-width grip. Start the lift by pushing the bar upward in a straight line to a position directly overhead—not in front of your body, but actually to a position in the same vertical plane as the middle of your head. Extend arms completely and pause at the top of the motion for a moment. Slowly, and under control, lower the bar to the starting position.

Tip: As you lift, when the bar passes your chin, tuck your chin to your chest to ensure proper posture. You want the bar to always be over your center of gravity and not forward or behind this point. Also, by tucking your chin, you will avoid looking up, which would cause you to arch your back and put you in a vulnerable position to be injured.

Rich Dalatri's NBA Strongmen

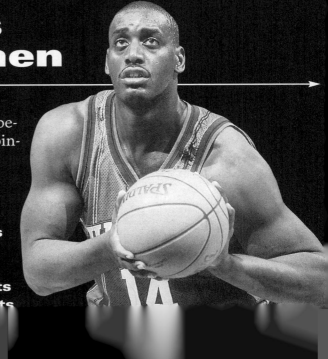

Here, with his twelve years of NBA experience, and in his admittedly subjective opinion, are the five strongest players in the NBA, pound for pound. Note that of the five, Dalatri has chosen two New Jersey Nets with whom he has worked.

1. **Jayson Williams, New Jersey Nets**
2. **Karl Malone, Utah Jazz**
3. **Alonzo Mourning, Miami Heat**
4. **Anthony Mason, Charlotte Hornets**
5. **Stephon Marbury, New Jersey Nets**

Ab Strength

Decline Medicine Ball Sit-Ups

Lying on a decline bench in the fully down position, hold a medicine ball in both hands with your arms extended overhead. Rise halfway as if you were going to throw the ball forward. Return slowly to the start position and repeat.

Put the medicine ball over the left shoulder, rise halfway on a diagonal motion to the right. Return slowly to the start position. Repeat the same motion for switching the ball to the right shoulder and rising on a diagonal path to the left.

Tip: If holding the ball overhead is too difficult, you may start with the ball on the chest and on the right and left shoulders as opposed to over the shoulders. Do all the prescribed repetitions for each position before moving to the next position.

Lower Back

Back Extension

On a back extension bench, start in a fully down position, with your face down and your hips on the pads. Position the pads of the bench so they rest at mid-thigh position. When you put the pads lower on the leg, you will work more hamstring than back. Put your hands behind your head. Rise to at least a parallel position to the floor. Hold the position for a one or two count and then slowly, under control, return to the start position. (When you become more experienced, this can be done with a weight held on the chest or behind the head.)

Tip: If you don't have access to a back extension bench, you can replicate the exercise on the floor. Lay facedown with your hands behind your head and rise upward so your chest and upper abdominal area is off the floor. Keep your toes in contact with the floor throughout the movement. Hold this up position for a one or two count, then lower slowly to the start position.

Legs

These exercises are for total leg development.

Squat

Start with your feet shoulder-width apart. Point the toes slightly outward. Place the bar on the top of the shoulders at the base of the neck. Grip the bar close to the shoulders. (By gripping the bar with this close grip, you ensure the chest and shoulders staying in a more upright position. By taking a wide grip, you allow the shoulders and chest to slump forward in a less favorable position.) Keep your back tight throughout the movement and your head in a neutral position.

From this position, lower the body under control by bending the knees and keeping the back straight and erect. Your heels never lose contact with the floor. Descend as if you are sitting in a chair. Keep your shins in a vertical position without pushing your knees forward. Descend to at least ninety degrees at the bottom of the motion for a moment. Never relax or bounce at the bottom position of the squat. Drive upward explosively to complete the lift.

Lunge

Place the bar on your shoulders at the base of your neck, feet in shoulder-width position. Take a long step forward. The foot placed forward should be far enough forward so when you are in a down (ninety-degree) position, your shin is in a vertical position and your knee is behind your foot, keeping the heel on the ground. The back foot rests on the toes throughout the exercise.

With the feet in proper position, bend the front leg at the knee. While descending, push the hips forward, keeping the back leg as straight as possible. The shoulders stay back behind the hips at all times and the chest remains out with the back straight. Keep head in a neutral position throughout the movement.

Descend to a ninety-degree angle in the front leg, pause for a moment, and then extend the front leg and come up to an erect position without moving your feet. Do the prescribed number of repetitions on one leg, then change legs. This exercise can also be performed using hand weights.

Tip: After becoming experienced in the lunge, you can also do it in a walking type of motion. Do one repetition on the right, then extend forward to do the next repetition on the left leg.

Weight Training

"Squats, bench press, cleans; lifts where you use the major muscle groups seem to be the most effective in gaining strength. That's the most important thing: not size, strength."

Brent Barry,
Seattle SuperSonics

If you were to ask ten experts what are the five most important strength training exercises for basketball players, you'd probably get ten completely different answers. Basketball players, like many athletes, need strength in a number of different areas of their bodies in order to be complete players.

- ***Strength in the stomach, back, and hips.*** These are the core muscles and they need to be strong to carry an athlete upright and help him handle the stress of repeatedly landing after jumping, as well as all the bumping and grinding that goes on in the battle for rebounds. All strength training exercises, which concentrate on these areas—with and without weights—would benefit a basketball player.

- ***Strength in the legs.*** Explosive types of lifts, as well as basic dynamic exercises such as running, jumping, and landing, are good for the hard-court athlete. If all else is equal, the player with strong legs will be able to outperform the player with average legs in the fourth quarter.

- ***Power movements.*** Quickness and agility are two of the most important aspects of a basketball player's game, and they can best be improved by adding strength up and down the body. Gaining lean muscle won't slow you down or make you any less agile. In fact, it will help you improve in both areas.

On the following pages are two **Explosive Exercises** recommended by Rich Dalatri.

For Basketball

LAMAR ODOM

61

Hang Clean (Lower Back/Hamstring/Shoulders)

Standing with your feet shoulder-width apart, grip the bar with a grip that puts your hands on the bar at a point just outside the width of your legs. Position the bar just above the knees, touching the thighs. Keep your back straight, but angled forward, your shoulders over the bar, and your knees bent slightly, keeping your head in a neutral position.

Start the pull by the active and explosive extension of the legs and back, driving the bar upward, following a straight path close to the body. As the legs and back extend, the arms then start to pull, and the elbows come upward and to the sides in the same vertical plane as the body. (Elbows cannot come forward or else the bar will move away from the body and not be in the straight line it needs to be in.) The body is completely extended, exploding upward in a jumplike position. When the pull is completed, immediately dip your body by bending your knees, and push your elbows forward under the bar, forcing the wrists to change to a catching position. The bar is caught over the center of gravity and not forward or backward, with feet flat on the floor. The change from pulling to catching must be quick or the bar will begin to drop, making it difficult to complete the lift.

Push Press (Shoulder)

Take the bar off the rack at shoulder level with a grip slightly wider than your shoulders. Place the bar on the upper front position of the shoulders. When the bar is resting here, do not relax the arms or shoulders.

Bend the knees about four inches. Keep the weight over your center of gravity and don't allow your knees to go in front of your feet and put you in a vulnerable position for injury. Explosively extend your legs, transferring the movement upward to the bar. The leg speed will initiate the upward movement on the bar by actively pushing it up. As the bar goes past your chin, tuck your chin to your chest to ensure you don't look up, making your head go backward, causing you to arch your back. (This could cause injury to your lower back.) The bar is pushed up until the arms are extended and the bar is fixed overhead in a position in the same plane as the middle of your head. (Do not push the bar forward.) If the bar is not resting on your shoulders when the leg drive is started, the speed generated from the legs cannot be fully transferred to the bar because the bar will first come down to the shoulders and then start upward, and most of the speed will have dissipated by this time.

Final Tip

Vary the workout.

"We never do the same workout twice," says Rich Dalatri of his Nets players. "You can change the weights, change the intensity, work on different body parts on different days. Change the exercises. Just do not do the same thing every day."

Rest

Recuperation and rest days are as important as the training itself. If you don't rest and let your body recuperate, you're not going to get the development you want.

Know your goals

Know what you want to achieve from your goals.

"Weight lifting gives me an advantage. I can lift and feel my physical presence in there. I use that in combination with the physical aspect of the game and it helps me prepare my game. It also helps me mentally and physically for the longevity and the long, grueling season."

Kevin Willis,
Toronto Raptors.

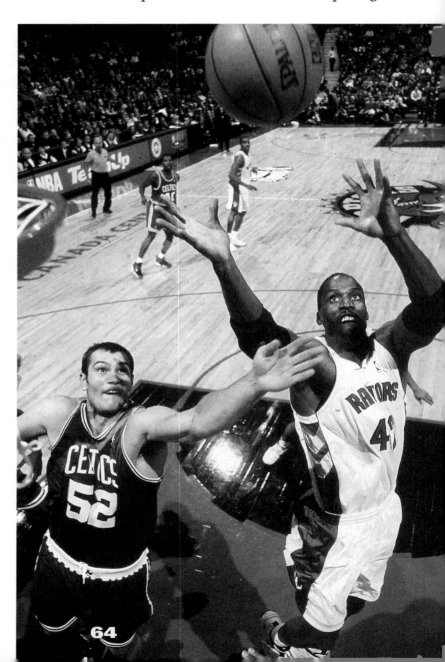

Chapter 4

The Care and Prevention of Athletic Injuries

TOM ABDENOUR

The first three chapters of this book discuss the upside of total fitness; how you will improve your health and overall physical well-being by following the routines and regimens we have illustrated. But there is a downside. With increased athletic activity also comes the possibility of injury. It's a reality in competitive sports; athletes get injured. But it is also a reality in weekend or casual athletic activity. The more you work out or compete in sports, the better the chance that you will experience some sort of injury. No matter how much you prepare yourself, there is no guarantee that you will be injury-free. Bad luck, unfortunately, sometimes wins out. If, however, you do experience an injury, there are ways to not only recover properly, but to speed up your recovery and get you back on the court sooner, rather than later.

Here are some of the more common sports-related injuries; their symptoms, description, care, and prevention.

65

Profile in Courage

After helping the University of Kansas capture the NCAA championship, Danny Manning was the NBA's number-one draft pick in 1988. In the twenty-sixth game of his rookie season with the Los Angeles Clippers, Manning suffered what is one of the worst knee injuries in athletics: he tore the anterior cruciate ligament (ACL) in his right knee. After surgery and rehab, Manning returned to play seventy or more games in each of the next four seasons. In 1995, after accepting a one-year contract with the Phoenix Suns, Manning suffered his second ACL injury, this one in his left knee. Despite the injury, he was rewarded with a six-year contract. Manning returned to the court in 1996 and 1997. But with just six games remaining in the 1997–98 season, Manning tore his right ACL again while making a hard cut under the basket in a game against the Sacramento Kings. It was the third such injury of his career.

One ACL injury can wipe out a career; three is an absolute death sentence. No player in any professional sport had ever come back from three ACL injuries. But Manning set out to prove the impossible. During the off-season, he worked extra hard on rehabilitating his knee, and was on the court for the opening of the 1998–99 season. He miraculously ended up playing in all fifty games of the shortened season. "Success isn't measured by the position you reach in life," Manning said. "Success in life is measured by the obstacles you overcome."

"Success isn't measured by the position you reach in life," Danny Manning said. "Success in life is measured by the obstacles you overcome."

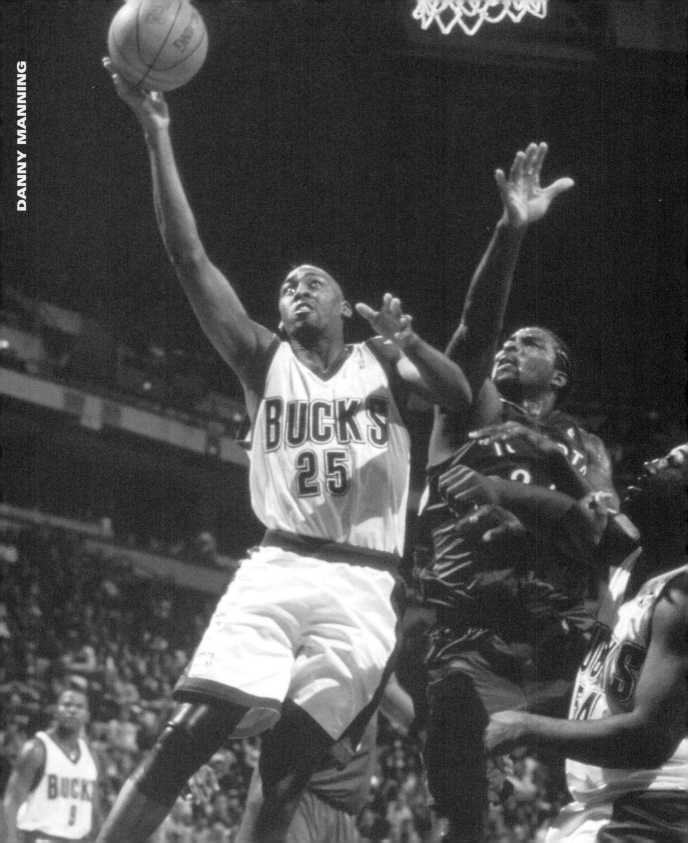

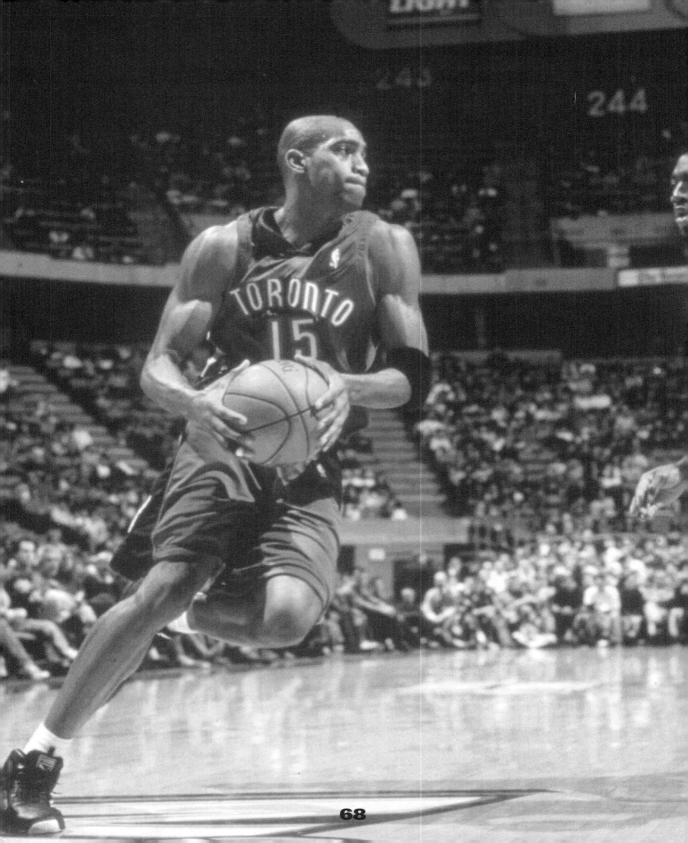

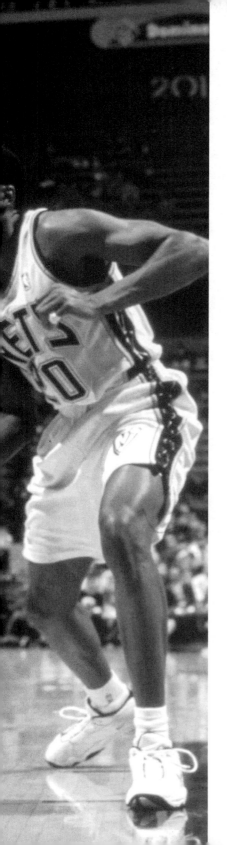

Meniscus Injuries

Knee Cartilage

Symptoms: Gradual pain on the inner side of the knee, buckling or giving out, can be signs of knee cartilage damage. If you have a locking in the joint, it could be caused by a torn portion of the meniscus catching on the end of the thighbone.

Description: This cartilage damage is usually caused by a severe twist of the knee, followed by the normal twisting and turning that occurs in most sports. The medial meniscus is the one most likely to be injured, but the lateral meniscus is also vulnerable to chronic wear and tear.

VINCE CARTER

Care: Follow the RICE procedures below and seek medical attention.

The acronym RICE is important to keep in mind whenever it comes to the care of musculoskeletal injuries. It stands for Rest, Ice, Compression, and Elevation, and can be used for bruises, dislocations, fractures, sprains, and strains.

Rest: You should stop moving your injured body part to avoid further injury and begin the healing process.

Ice: Protecting the skin with a wet elastic bandage or wet towel, an ice pack should be applied as quickly as possible to the injured area for twenty to thirty minutes every two to three hours during the first 24 to 48 hours following the injury. Once the area becomes numb, temporarily remove the ice pack to avoid possible frostbite or nerve damage. The cold helps reduce swelling by constricting the blood vessels in the injured area, dulling the pain and relieving muscle spasms as well. Crushed ice is best, but cubes will do. The ice should be placed in a double plastic bag, hot water bottle, or wet towel.

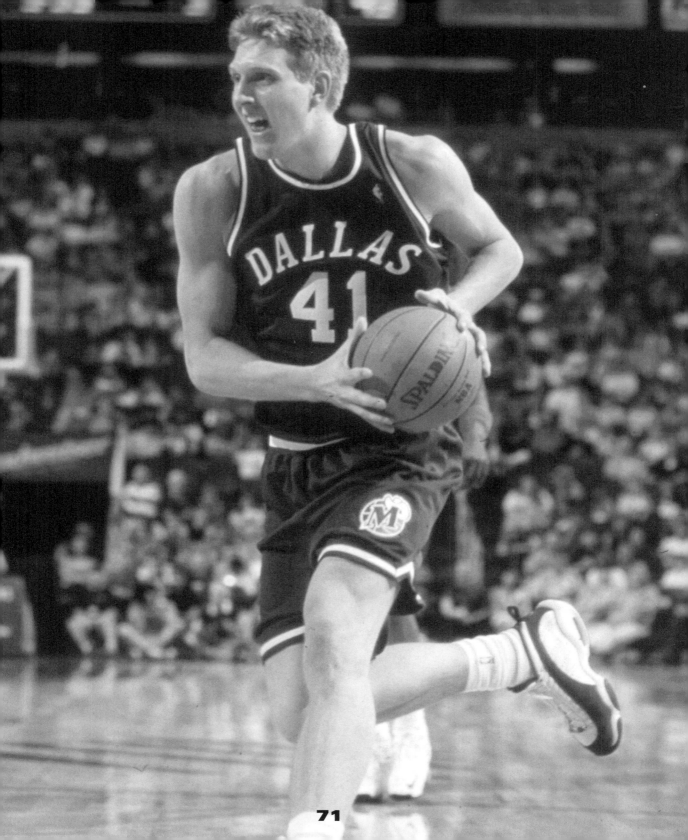

Compression: Apply a wet elastic bandage to the injured area for compression, which may squeeze some fluid and debris out of the injury site, limit internal bleeding, and protect the skin from the ice pack. Start the bandage below the injury by several inches and wrap in an upward, overlapping manner until several inches above the injury. Stretch the elastic bandage to approximately seventy percent of its capacity for proper compression and leave the fingers and toes exposed. This surface layer bandage should be kept on the injury for 18 to 24 hours. Once you've applied the ice pack, wrap another elastic bandage over the ice to hold it in place.

Elevation: Elevation of the injured area limits circulation, internal bleeding, and swelling. Make sure the injured area is above the level of the heart whenever possible for the first 24 hours following the injury. But if a fracture is suspected, do not elevate an extremity until it has been stabilized with a splint. Some fractures should not be elevated at all.

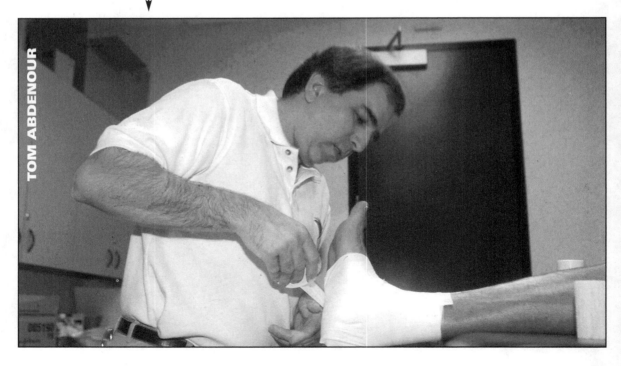

TOM ABDENOUR

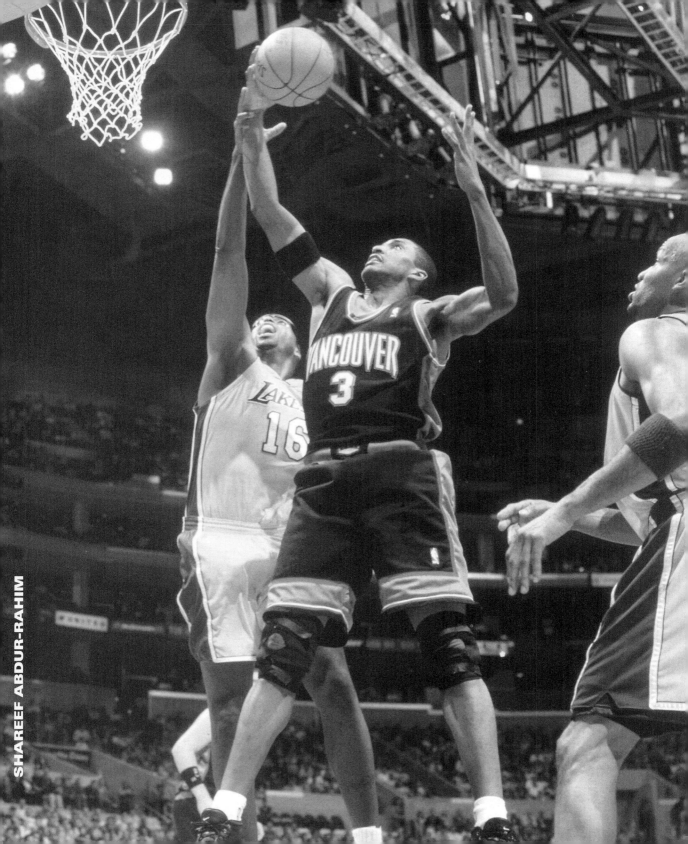

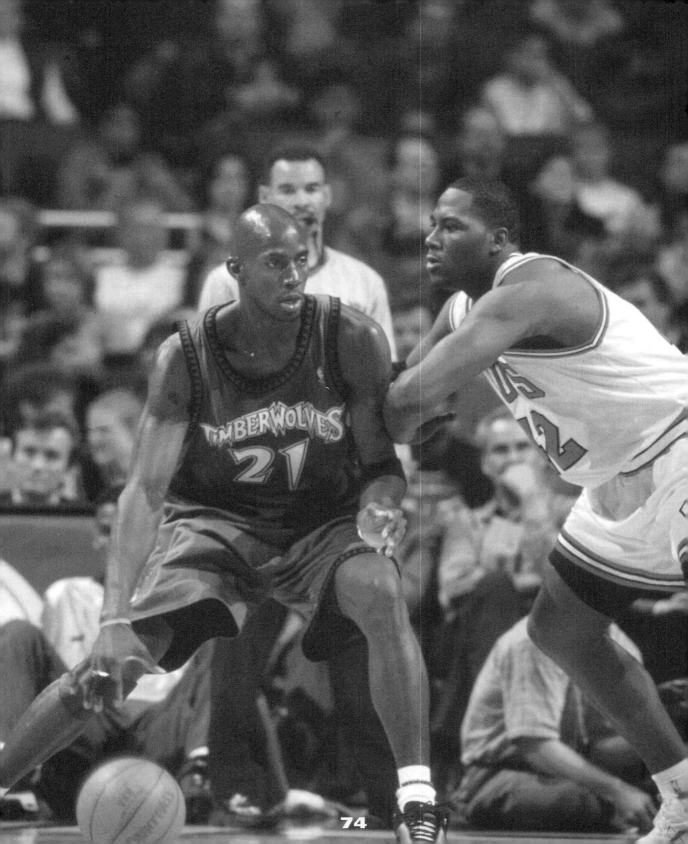

74

Shoulder Separation

Symptoms: Ligament damage, which can range from mild to severe, will result in a bump at the shoulder tip, which will be very tender to the touch and painful with movement, especially forward and sideways.

Description: By putting your fingers on the tip of the shoulder, you can tell that this is a vulnerable area because it is not well-padded. A direct hit to this area, caused either by another player or from falling on the floor, can cause ligament damage severe enough to result in the bones of the joint separating from each other. This is a combination of a contusion and a sprain.

Care: If you suspect that you've separated your shoulder, you need to seek medical attention immediately. While you're waiting for that help to arrive, put your arm into a sling and carefully apply a cold pack.

KEVIN GARNETT VS. ELTON BRAND

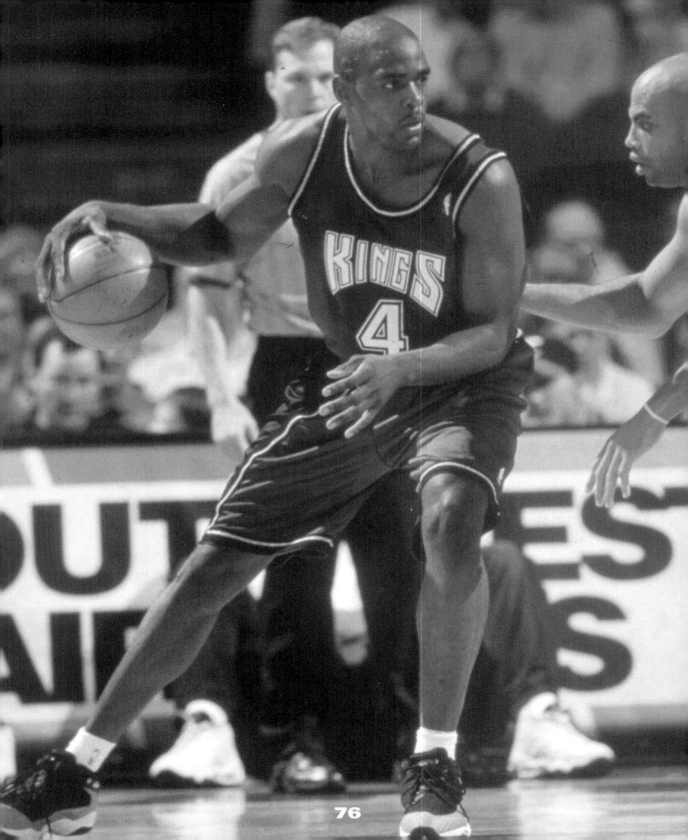

If you're looking for a shoulder to cry on, don't ask Chris Webber. The Sacramento Kings forward has had his share of shoulder problems, but has battled through them without asking for sympathy. The shoulder may not be one of the most frequently injured body parts for basketball players, but the injuries that do occur in this area can be just as debilitating as those to more commonly injured areas. Webber is an example of a player who has come back from two serious shoulder injuries.

He originally dislocated his right shoulder as a member of the Washington Bullets (now Wizards) during the 1994–95 season by diving to save a loose ball and landing on his outstretched arm, forcing the humeral bone out of its socket. After the bone was put back into place, Webber's arm was put into a sling and the shoulder was iced regularly.

Since the labrum was not torn and the ligaments appeared to be fine, surgery was not recommended. While he was out for six weeks, Webber rehabbed with active and passive range-of-motion exercises, strengthening with light weights and gradually giving way to heavier weights, electrical stimulation, ultrasound, massage, and exercise on a UBE (upper body ergometer), which is like pedaling a bike upside down.

CHRIS WEBBER

> "They say that once this type of surgery is performed, your teeth will come out before your shoulder does," Washington Wizards head athletic trainer Kevin Johnson says.

"With the combination of Chris's dedication to his rehab and our aggressiveness as a medical staff, Chris had an above-normal recovery," says Wizards head athletic trainer, Kevin Johnson. "But once you've suffered a shoulder separation, the likelihood of it recurring increases due to the muscles and tendons being weaker. And that's what happened with Chris."

Webber suffered another right shoulder dislocation the following season (1995–96), and because of the pronounced weakness of the muscles and tendons in that area, he missed the rest of the season. A type of surgery called the Bankart repair, in which the muscles are tightened to the humeral head of the bone, was performed.

"They say that once this type of surgery is performed, your teeth will come out before your shoulder does," Johnson says.

Webber returned to play for the Wizards in 1996–97 with no recurrence of the injury. He was traded to the Kings in May 1998, where he shouldered much of the responsibility of leading the team to a playoff berth and a near first-round upset of Utah in 1999.

Elbow Injuries
Bursitis

Symptoms: A swollen bursa sac will hang from the bottom of the elbow and may feel warm and tender. The fluid can affect elbow range of motion.

Description: Located at the tip of the elbow, the bursa sac is normally filled with a lubricating fluid for the elbow joint. Falling on your elbow can inflame this sac.

Care: A bruised bursa sac usually doesn't become swollen until the next day, so if you banged this area hard enough for it to hurt, apply a cold pack three to four times a day.

Tennis Elbow

Symptoms: Ongoing pain, usually felt when using your arm in a swinging motion, is located over the bony point at the side of the elbow.

Description: Repeated stress to the forearm muscles causes inflammation of the tendon that goes from the muscles on top of the forearm to the bony knob on the outside of the elbow.

Care: Use an ice pack for thirty minutes following activity. Ask your physician to recommend a rehabilitation program.

Wrist Sprain and Fracture

Symptoms: If you have pain when moving your wrist, followed by swelling and bruising, you may have a sprain or fracture. Grip strength and flexibility in the wrist will be affected.

Description: The backward bending of the hand, especially in a fall or a collision with another athlete, can stretch or tear a ligament around the wrist.

Care: If moving your wrist is painful after applying an ice pack for thirty minutes, seek medical attention. Both a serious sprain and a fracture need medical treatment.

Allan Houston, whose superb shooting helped the New York Knicks reach the 1999 NBA Finals, has overcome a serious right wrist injury that required rehabilitative surgery. One of the ways that Houston strengthens his wrist is by swinging and catching a bright orange medicine ball that hangs from the ceiling of the Knick's weight room.

ALLAN HOUSTON

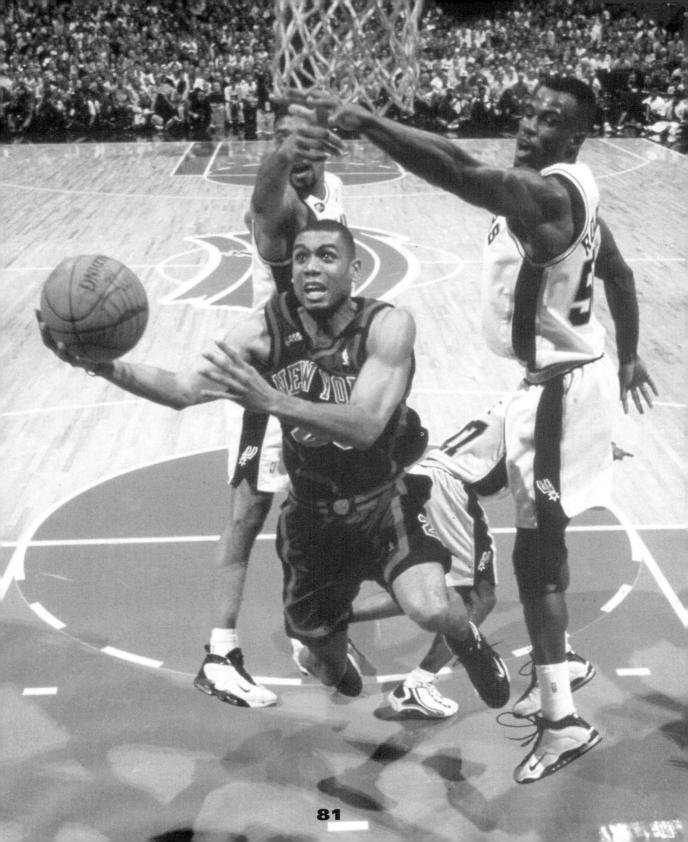

Foot Injuries
Stress Fractures

Symptoms: The pain comes from the site of a bump over the bone, occurring during and after activity.

Description: Repeated jumping and running subjects bones to impact, which can cause a series of microfractures in various bones of the foot.

Care: Apply an ice pack for twenty to thirty minutes, then obtain a medical evaluation before returning to play. If there is no fracture, taping the area can help support it.

Bone Spurs/Heel Spurs

Symptoms: If you've experienced a recent change in your activity such as running more often or greater distances, you may get pain at the bottom of your heel. This pain is often worse while running and in the morning.

Description: With this injury you'll have inflammation of the plantar fascia, which is the thick fibrous tissue that runs the length of the long arch on the sole of the foot and attaches to dhe heel bone.

Care: Apply ice three or four times a day. Deeply massaging the foot will also help, especially in the morning.

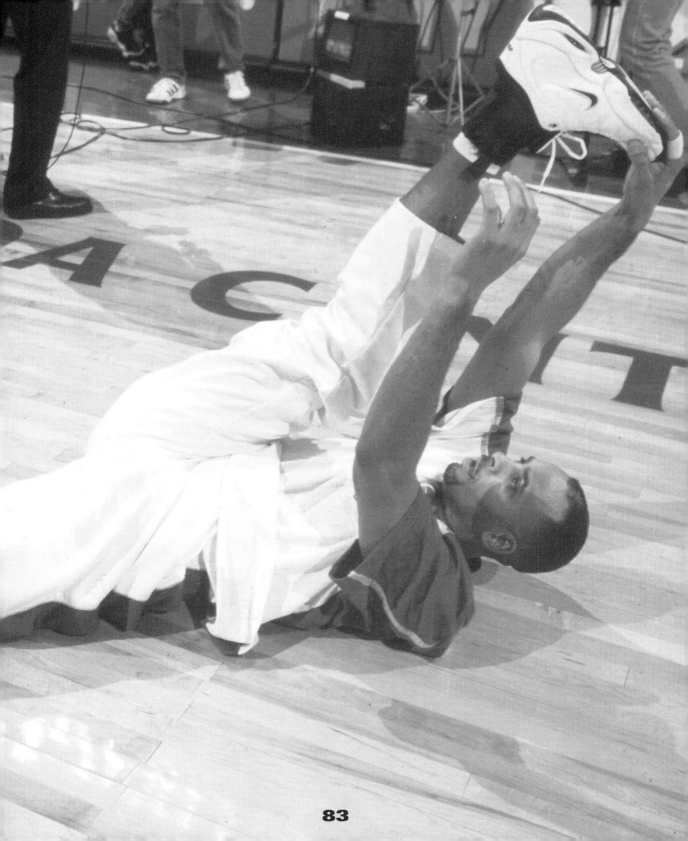

Ways to Help Prevent Thece Injuries

Meniscus Injuries: The best preventative for this type of injury is building strength and flexibility in the area surrounding the knee joint with regular exercises.

Shoulder Separation: When you're falling onto the ground, especially on a hardwood floor, try to roll into the fall rather than land directly on the tip of the shoulder.

Elbow Injuries (Bursitis): Wear an elbow pad while playing if you're vulnerable to this type of injury.

Elbow Injuries (Tennis Elbow): Strengthen and stretch the muscles in your shoulder and arm. Use a heating pad on the area prior to activity.

Wrist Sprain and Fracture: Strengthen and stretch the muscles in your forearm and wrist. Practice falling in a tuck and roll manner to avoid falling directly on your hand and rolling over it.

Foot Injuries (Stress Fractures/Bone Spurs/ Heel Spurs): Find athletic shoes that give you as much cushion and arch support as possible to soften the impact when running and jumping.

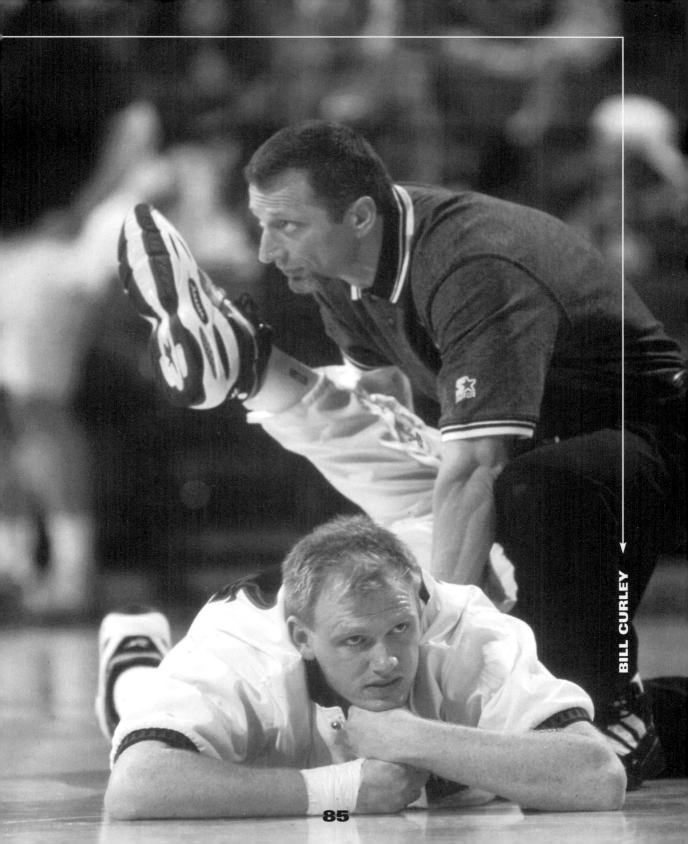

BILL CURLEY

Basketball-Related

You've seen it at least a hundred times. An NBA player grimaces with pain after injuring an ankle, a knee, his back, a hamstring, or his groin area. You can feel his pain. Why? Because you've probably done the same thing yourself more times than you'd care to remember. Maybe it's only a temporary irritation and you can bounce back quickly. Or maybe it's more serious and you have to come out of the game or even miss some playing time as a result. No two injuries are exactly alike, but there are some common features of injuries to specific parts of your body.

The following sections are designed to help you identify the most common basketball-related injuries—ankle sprain and fracture, jumper's knee, low back strain/soreness, hamstring muscle strain, and groin muscle strain—as well as to learn the proper procedures to deal with these setbacks in order to put you back on the court as quickly—and safely—as possible.

Injuries

LATRELL SPREWELL

Profile in Courage II

Are there any doubts that the ankle is the number-one culprit for basketball-related injuries? Listen to the Kurt Thomas story. Thomas, who now plays for the New York Knicks, has had five ankle fractures (three to his right ankle, two to his left). In February 1997, as a member of the Dallas Mavericks, Thomas's right ankle was in a cast, healing from a previous injury. Soon after he returned to action, he refractured the same ankle, and had surgery in May 1997. He recovered, but in November 1997 he fractured the right ankle yet again. This time, however, he opted against surgery after consulting with specialists and the Dallas team doctor.

Roger Hinds, the head athletic trainer of the Dallas Mavericks, remembers how he treated Thomas. "We placed him in a weight-bearing boot brace for protection while he was healing," Hinds recalls. "The lockout of 1998 extended the layoff and helped give him more time to heal. He also reduced his body weight to about 230 to 235, down from 250." Time and the boot brace finally healed the ankle, and Thomas contributed to the Knick's amazing 1999 playoff run.

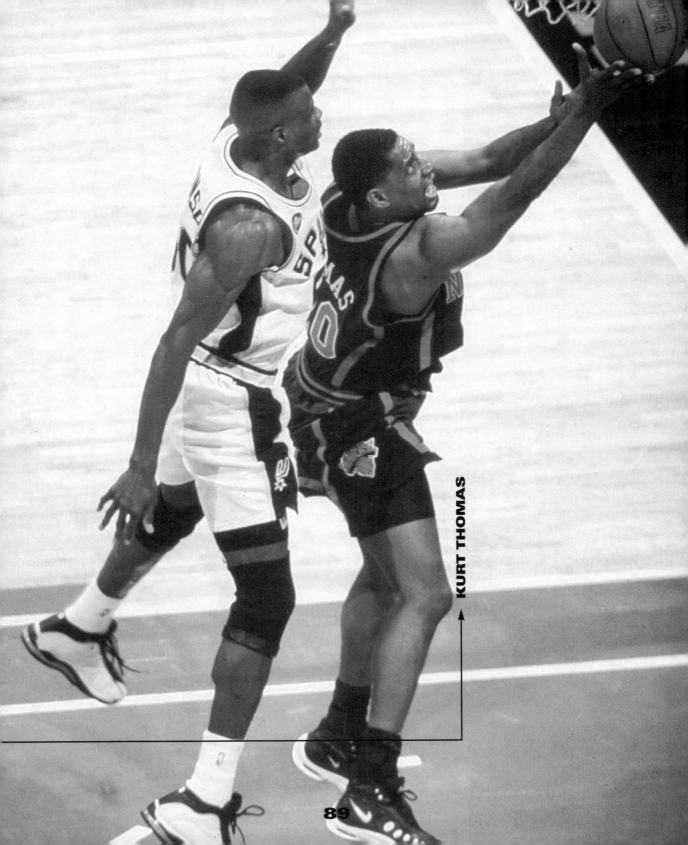

KURT THOMAS

89

Ankle Sprain/Fracture

Symptoms: With an ankle sprain or fracture, you'll experience immediate pain, often accompanied by a tearing or "popping" feeling, plus difficulty in walking. You'll also get swelling and tenderness in the area very quickly. If you have difficulty with weight bearing, it could indicate a fracture or a significant sprain.

Description: An ankle sprain is the result of one or more of the ligaments holding the bones of the ankle joint together stretching, tearing, or rupturing. Approximately 85 percent of ankle sprains involve the outside (lateral) ligaments and are caused by having the ankle turned or twisted inward. Fractures can occur the same way.

Care: Remove your shoe and sock quickly. Use an elastic wrap to cover the ankle and to hold a pack of crushed ice, which should be applied for twenty to thirty minutes every two to three hours over the next 48 hours. Keep the ankle elevated as much as possible until the swelling is gone. If you think you may have a fracture, use crutches or a cane to support walking, if possible, until examined by a physician.

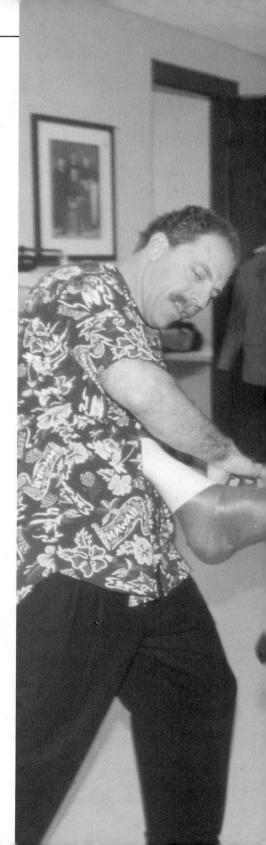

SHAQUILLE O'NEAL BEING TAPED BY TRAINER

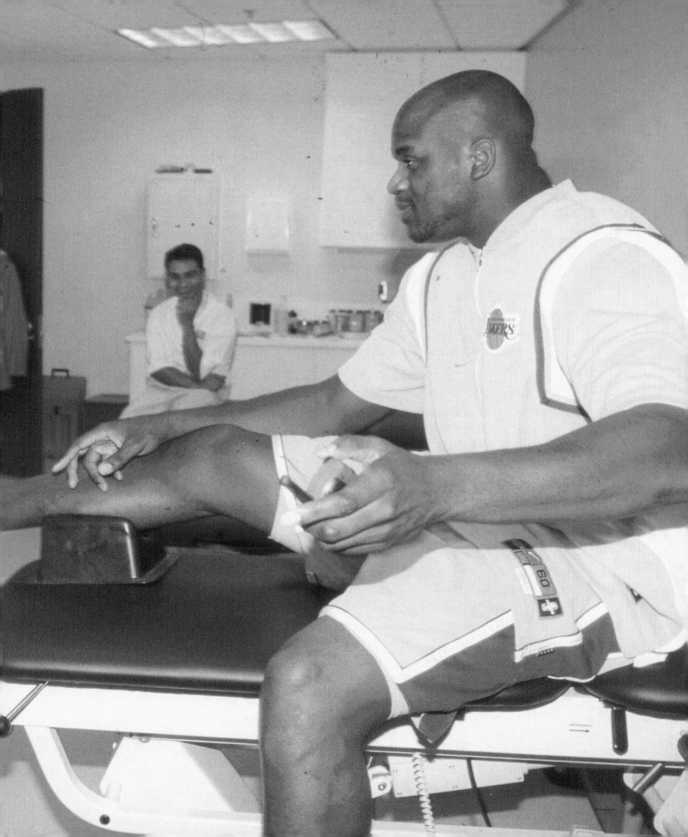

"Jumper's Knee"

Symptoms: Very few sports involve more jumping than basketball, so it's not surprising to see this injury in the top five. Gradual pain from "jumper's knee" occurs just below the kneecap, and is often felt when you're sitting or when straightening your leg after you've been jumping or running.

Description: The inflammation of the tendon that attaches the kneecap to the tibia is caused by a strain on the ligament in sports involving jumping, such as basketball. It's one of the most common overuse injuries in all of sports.

Care: As with many other overuse injuries, jumper's knee will benefit from some heat before the activity and cold afterward. The heat can be in the form of a heating pad, hot water bottle, or Jacuzzi type of hot tub. Also, there are many neoprene rubber knee sleeves and other supports that can provide relief. After the activity, use a cold pack or ice massage. If the case is severe, the best option may be rest.

The patella—better known as the kneecap—lies in front of the hinge joint formed by the femur and tibia. The patella tendon connects the patella to the tibial tuberosity, and acts as a shock absorber. The constant pressure produced by running and jumping is what causes the tendon to become inflamed.

Among the many basketball players who suffer from patellar tendinitis is Sacramento Kings forward Corliss Williamson, who wears a thin band underneath his left knee that puts pressure on the tendon to deflect pain away from this joint, and helps relieve the stress of jumping.

The Kings strength and conditioning coach, Al Biancani, works with Williamson to support his knee by strengthening his quadriceps. Stronger quads relieve the strain on the patellar tendon and reduce the inflammation.

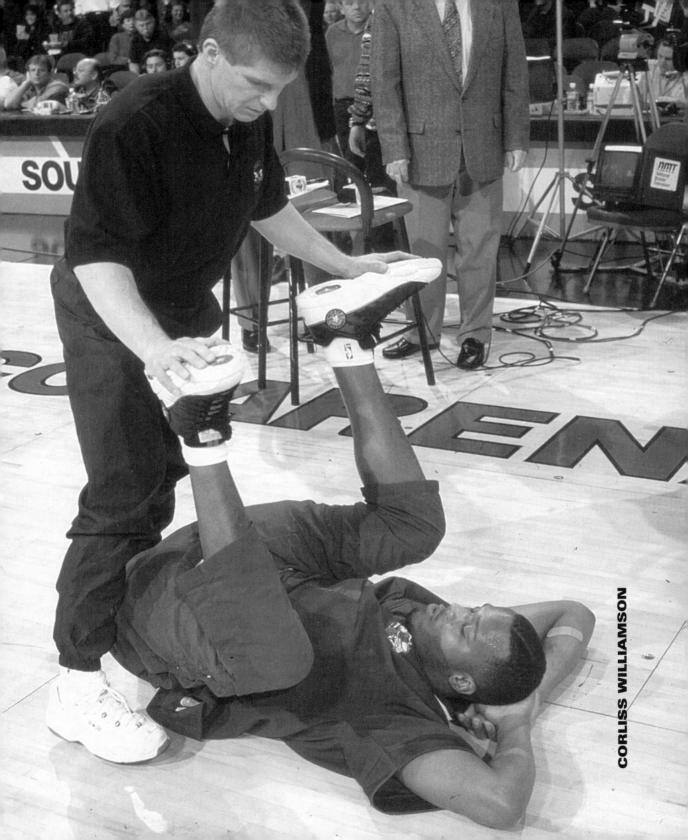

CORLISS WILLIAMSON

Low Back Strain/Soreness

Symptoms: Almost every athlete knows the pain associated with low back strain and soreness. The symptoms range from low grade pain and stiffness in the lower back to piercing pain accompanied by spasms. Movements—especially bending—may be limited.

Description: Overuse of muscles during activities such as bending down or lifting objects causes inflammation of one or more of the back muscles or ligaments.

Care: Apply an ice pack for the first two or three days after the onset of pain, then gently stretch the area. Once you've returned to the court, ice the area after activity. Chronic back pain is miserable, so get medical attention for a rehabilitation program.

SHAQUILLE O'NEAL

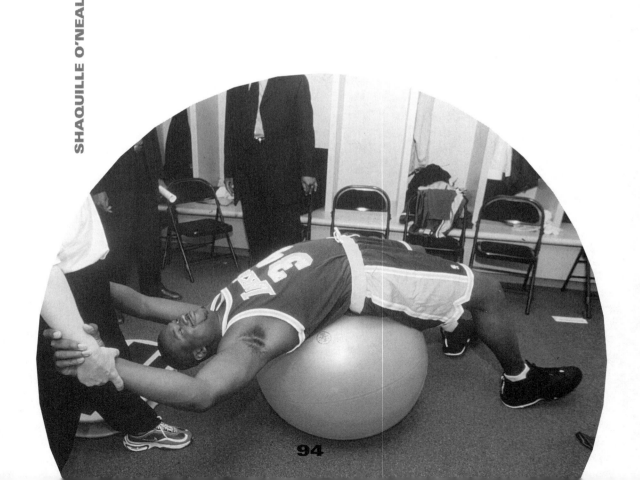

Hamstring Muscle Strain ←

Symptoms: As with most injuries, the severity of a hamstring strain can vary greatly. You may feel anything from a pull to a severe pain behind your thigh, usually when sprinting. Tenderness, swelling, and either stiffness or pain will follow.

Description: Hamstring strain will occur when one or more of the three hamstring muscles is stretched or torn by a contraction of the hamstring muscles when you accelerate while running. Sometimes it can result from an imbalance of power between the quadriceps and the hamstrings.

Care: Follow the RICE procedures (see page 70). Wrap a compression pad under an elastic bandage and apply it to the hamstring area. During the first night's sleep following the injury, you should be woken to gently stretch the injured muscle.

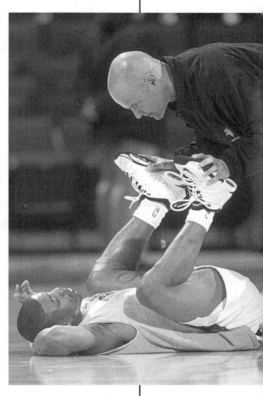

TYRONE "MUGGSY" BOGUES

Groin Muscle Strain

Symptoms: One of the most debilitating of injuries, the groin muscle strain comes on as a sudden, sharp pain in the groin, and continues with pain when you're trying to draw your leg inward. The pain may be followed by tenderness, swelling, and bruising.

Description: This injury is a stretch or a tear of the muscle that runs from the pubic bone to the inside of the thigh, which can occur when you make a sudden switch in direction or when you twist your thigh with your legs spread apart.

Care: Wrap a compression bandage with a pad over the area. Apply an ice pack for twenty to thirty minutes three to four times a day for two days. You should also stretch the area in a slow, pain-free manner. As with the hamstring strain, you should be woken to gently stretch the injured muscle during the first night's sleep following the injury.

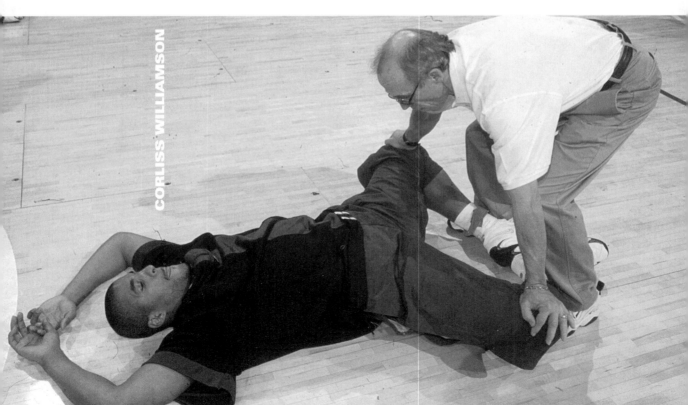

CORLISS WILLIAMSON

Five Ways to Prevent Basketball Injuries

No matter how careful you are, some athletic injuries are inevitable. But there are steps you can take that will lessen the likelihood of getting hurt and having to sit on the sidelines while your friends are out there competing. Golden State Warriors head athletic trainer Tom Abdenour offers five ways to prevent injuries on the basketball court:

1. Ankle Support: Be sure to minimize your chances of sustaining an ankle sprain by using an external support, such as an ankle brace, or tape your ankle. Not only will ankle support reduce your chances of being injured, it will minimize the severity of a sprain if one occurs.

2. Keep Your Knee Strong and Flexible: A strong knee is less likely to sustain certain acute or overuse injuries, such as jumper's knee. Flexible quadriceps muscles also are important in the prevention of overuse injuries. Here is a simple way to assess this: lie on your stomach and bend your knee back as much as possible. Grab your ankle and pull it back even farther. The closer your heel comes to your buttocks, the more flexibility you possess. Compare one knee to the other, and if there is a difference, you should spend some time stretching the less flexible leg.

TOM ABDENOUR

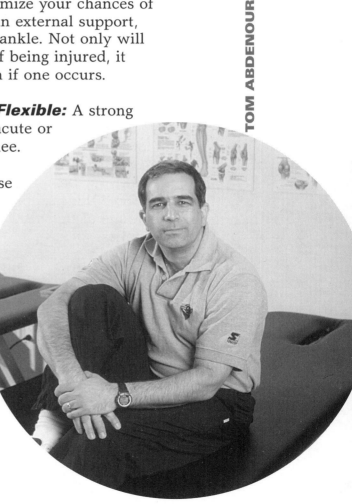

3. Pay Attention to Pain in the Achilles, Kneecap, and Hamstring:
If there is pain from tendinitis in the Achilles and kneecap, or a hamstring strain, rest is needed. Don't force your way through some of these pains. Let the inflammation settle, then strengthen the area before resuming activities.

4. Maintain Flexibility in the Low Back:
Don't neglect flexibility for the low back. It is vulnerable to stress from sprains, strains, and contusions. If you have a chronic back ailment, stick with a good rehabilitation program that will allow you to enhance your cardiovascular fitness through basketball.

5. Lifting Weights for Your Upper Body Will Not Affect Your Shot:
A good upper body strength training program will help prevent shoulder and arm injuries (see Chapter 3). Balance this work with stretching exercises to maintain your flexibility. If you need a role model to reinforce this premise, just look to Chris Mullin, one of the NBA's best pure shooters of the nineties.

"Every NBA player is different, of course, but one thing that some of the best have in common is how they approach rehabilitation from an injury," says Golden State Warriors head athletic trainer Tom Abdenour. "None of them sit around feeling sorry for themselves when they're hurt. Instead, they approach rehab with the same vigor as they do competition in a game. I've worked with some of the NBA's best players who have sustained assorted season-ending injuries, such as Chris Mullin and Tim Hardaway. Each of these players approached his rehabilitation with a competitive, positive mental attitude, knowing each day that went by represented one day closer to resuming full activity.

"It is important to set meaningful goals that can be reached within the medical parameters of the injury. Examples of time frames are: when you can return strong enough to shoot jump shots, when you can run the length of the floor, when you can play one-on-one, etc. These types of goals are great benchmarks to keep you focused and motivated to complete the sometimes arduous and tedious rehabilitation process. Goal setting, positive reinforcement, and keeping a focus on a return to play are all vital components of the best approach to restoring an injury to full strength, both mentally and physically."

Profile in Courage III

Wherever New York Knicks center Chris Dudley goes, he carries a small black box with him. In the box are needles and insulin. Chris Dudley has diabetes. He has had the disease since he was a teenager. Diabetes starts when the pancreas no longer produces insulin, the hormone that regulates the metabolism of glucose and other carbohydrates. The insulin is needed to balance the blood-sugar levels in the body. If the balance is off, the result can be anything from dizziness to a coma. To regulate the disease, a diabetic must constantly watch his or her blood sugar levels and administer injections of insulin to keep that fragile balance. He is the only known player in the NBA to have the disease.

"You have to know your own body; you have to be your own doctor," Dudley says. And what makes it so demanding is that the disease is with him all the time. "You can't take a break. You always have it. It's not like you can work out hard for a week and then take a week off. You have to deal with diabetes constantly."

Dealing with it is what Dudley does. That means four insulin injections daily into his right or left thigh and constant testing of his blood-sugar levels, including one at half-time of every game. So, along with the assortment of bumps and bruises any NBA player endures, Dudley has a heavier burden to bear. But as Chris Dudley's wife, Christine, says, he has never let the disease stop him from playing the game he loves. "Chris is incredibly tolerant to adversity. He plays through pain. There are no excuses."

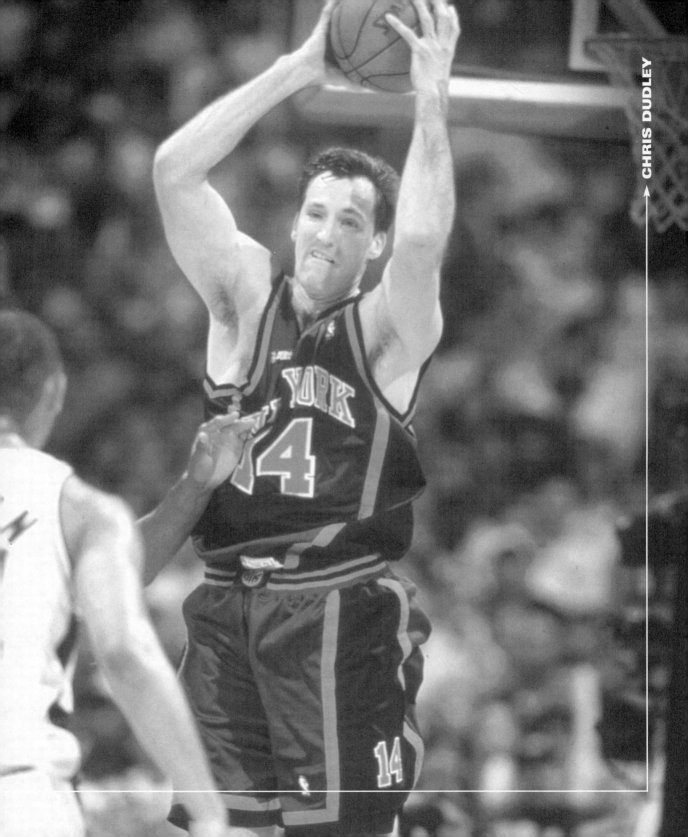
CHRIS DUDLEY

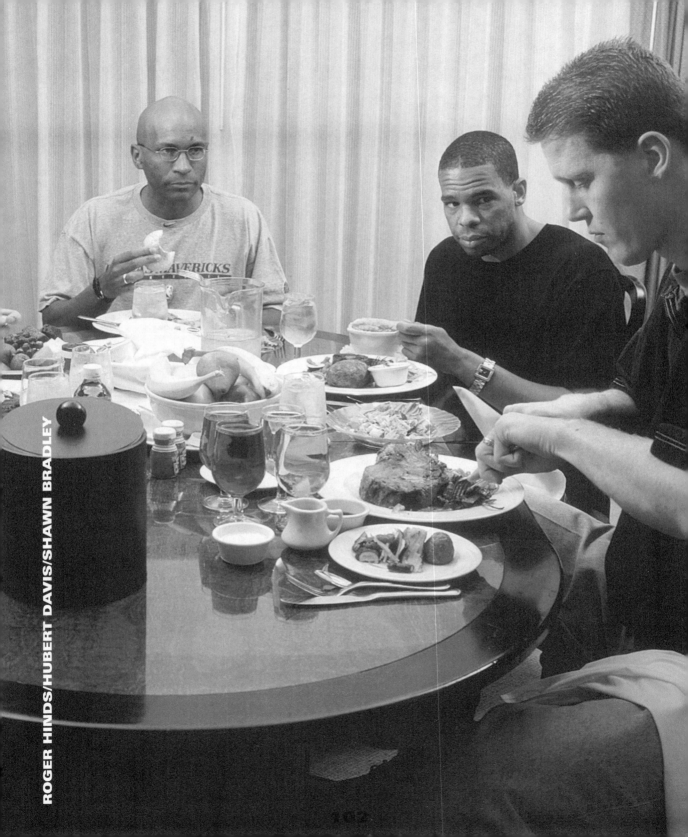

Chapter 5

Nutrition

Remember that old saying, "You are what you eat"? It's true.

Even in the NBA, where players have the best facilities, guidance, and support available, players still sometimes fall prey to a poor diet and its consequences. Some have paid dearly for such transgressions—with their careers. So, following all the good advice given in the previous four chapters of this book and then neglecting your diet and proper nutrition is a recipe for failure. You can do all the lifting, stretching, and cardiovascular training in the world, but if you don't eat right, achieving total fitness will still remain just an elusive goal.

Roger Hinds, the head athletic trainer of the Dallas Mavericks, recollects the sad story of one player, who shall remain nameless. "This guy has all but eaten himself out of the league," Hinds says. "When he played for us, we'd tell him what to eat, and he wouldn't listen to us. It just didn't matter to him. We told him if he dropped fifty pounds, he'd be a better player, and he'd be a healthier player.

"But he ate whatever he wanted,

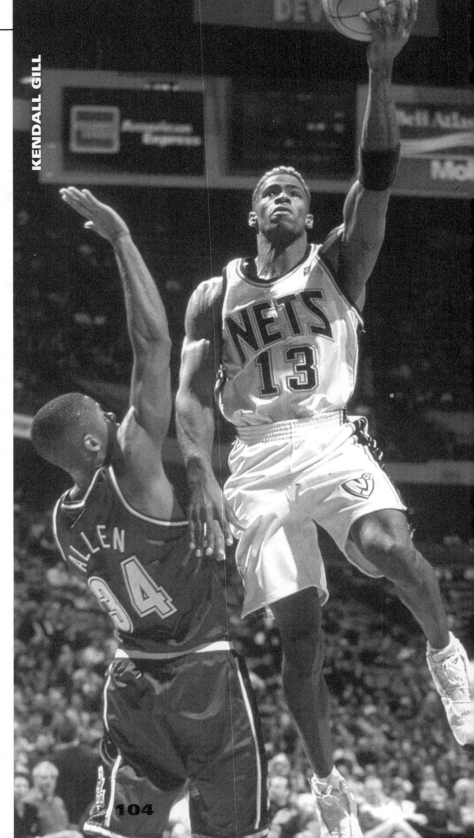

KENDALL GILL

"I'm realizing more and more that if good nutrition can make or break a bodybuilder, then it isn't very hard to believe that better nutrition will also help a pro basketball player. And I need every edge to stay one step ahead of the competition. I don't carry as much fat on my body as I used to.

whenever he wanted. Some teams he played for sent him to fat farms, and he'd lose weight, but in a couple of months he'd put it all back on. It got to the point where people would just throw up their hands with him. It's one of the saddest cases I've ever seen."

Hinds remembered another player who had a weight clause written into his contract, but that didn't have much effect, since people would sneak him food at night during training camp.

Tragic tales, yes. But not every story involving an NBA player's love of food has a sad ending.

"I'd say about sixty percent of the players in the league are cognizant of what they eat," Hinds notes, "especially the veterans. When they start to realize their bodies are beginning to wear out, they start to get on a health kick.

"The young guys, however, are different. They're so used to eating fast food, and you can't eat that kind of stuff and sustain the level of energy you need to compete at this level. When I was in Atlanta, every time we'd see one of our guys bringing fast food back to the hotel on the road, they got fined. But that didn't really stop them. They'd just have the cab drivers drive them around while they ate, so we wouldn't see them. But the older guys are a lot more careful with what they eat.

"The young kids will listen to you talk about what they should be eating, but a lot of them get caught up in all these fads. They'll come up to me and show me some kind of energy bar made of tree bark or something, and I'll say to them, 'You want to eat a tree? Go out and chew on one instead of spending all your money on something that hasn't been tested and may not do you any good.'"

Hinds sums up the body's need for the right kinds of food with an appropriate analogy.

"I used to own a 1981 Corvette Classic Anniversary model with 350 horsepower and a four-barrel carburetor," he says. "I loved that car and usually gave it the best treatment I could. When I would use 93 octane gasoline, it ran like a charm and I received considerable enjoyment from it. But if I'd skimp and put 87 octane into it, the engine would start knocking and performance would drop noticeably.

I'm stronger and more explosive to the basket. I can hold my position on the court. I'm lighter now and just as able to dominate my opponent at a lighter weight."
Kendall Gill, New Jersey Nets

"Well, our bodies are similar. We can't keep putting the wrong fuels into our tanks if we expect to perform at our best. No matter what sport you compete in, you need to eat right in order to perform better. And athletes who maintain a proper diet—in combination with strength training, stretching, cardiovascular exercise, and proper injury prevention—recover more quickly between performances and avoid injuries caused by fatigue.

"Simply put, if all else is equal, the athlete who controls his food and beverage intake will outperform the athlete who doesn't."

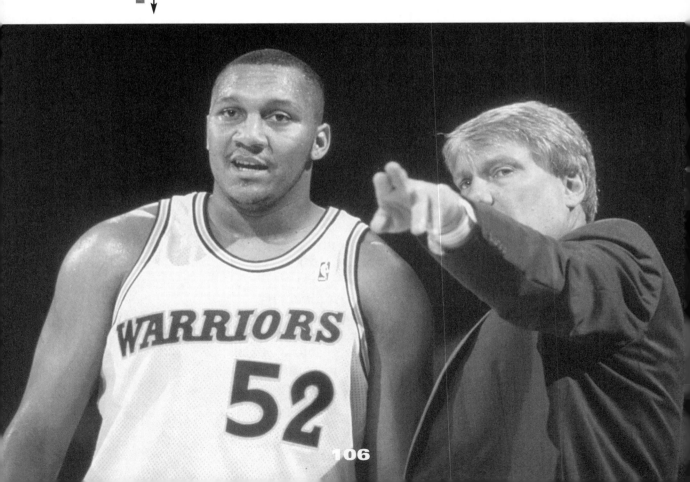

The Diet Police

A well-documented story from a few seasons back featured Victor Alexander, formerly of the Golden State Warriors. Don Nelson, a food lover himself, who coached the Warriors at the time, was wandering through the kitchen of the hotel where the team was staying. A call came for room service, ordering three hamburgers. The call came from Alexander's room.

Knowing Alexander had to make a certain weight the following day or face a fine, Nelson had an idea.

A short time later, Alexander answered the door to his room, and immediately lost his appetite. There was Nelson, who had put on a waiter's jacket and delivered the burgers himself. Alexander first tried to stammer there had been some mistake, but Nelson just walked away after telling his player to enjoy his meal, knowing full well he'd be accepting fine money the following day.

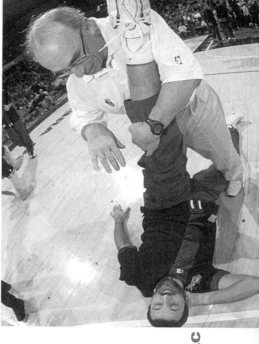

VLADE DIVAC

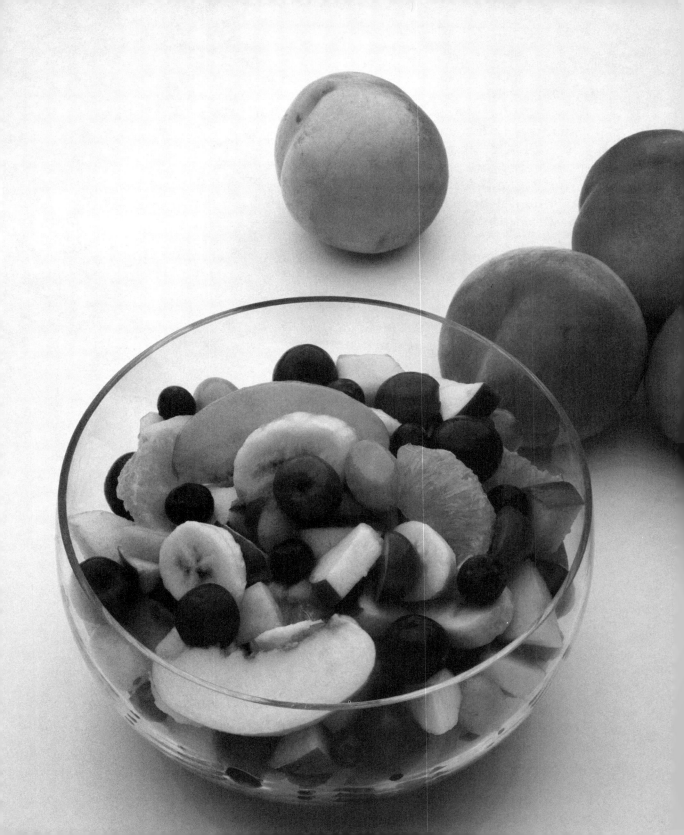

Good Nutrition

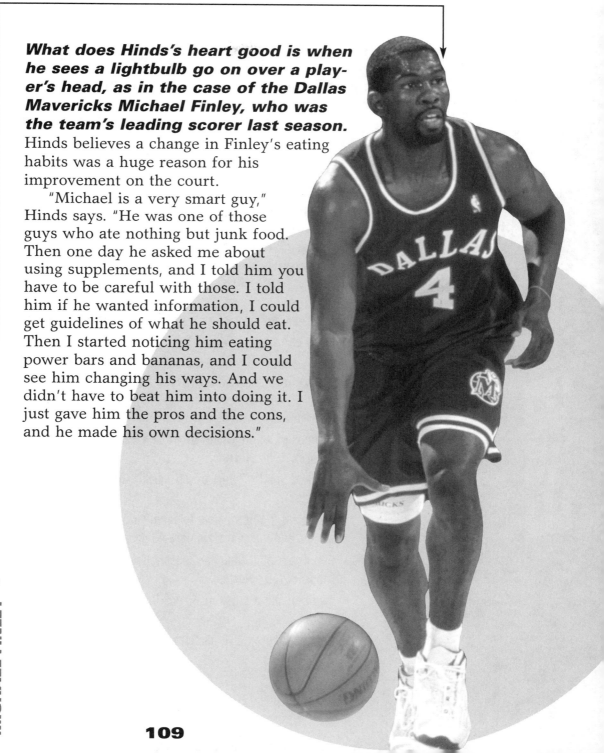

What does Hinds's heart good is when he sees a lightbulb go on over a player's head, as in the case of the Dallas Mavericks Michael Finley, who was the team's leading scorer last season. Hinds believes a change in Finley's eating habits was a huge reason for his improvement on the court.

"Michael is a very smart guy," Hinds says. "He was one of those guys who ate nothing but junk food. Then one day he asked me about using supplements, and I told him you have to be careful with those. I told him if he wanted information, I could get guidelines of what he should eat. Then I started noticing him eating power bars and bananas, and I could see him changing his ways. And we didn't have to beat him into doing it. I just gave him the pros and the cons, and he made his own decisions."

MICHAEL FINLEY

Despite the best intentions of everyone, old habits die hard. One such case is that of A.C. Green, who came to the Mavericks in a trade with Phoenix, and immediately saw his playing time increase substantially from what he was used to.

"A.C. just didn't want to eat before practices," Hinds says, "but he found he wasn't able to play at the level he was accustomed to if he didn't. So he'd get up early, eat breakfast, and go back to bed. Then he'd get up and go to practice."

Not that such a routine is recommended, but the best advice is: lay off fats and cholesterol. Be wary of nutritional fads. Drink plenty of water, about eight glasses a day. Stick with lean meats, plenty of fruits and vegetables, and make sure you start the day with a good breakfast.

Roger Hinds's Recommended Pregame Meal

This meal is designed for a six-foot-one, 195-pound athlete. It is a high-carbohydrate, low-fat meal that should be consumed four to five hours before activity. Total calories are approximately 700.

- 2 slices of whole wheat bread and 2 tablespoons of grape jelly (approx. 120 calories)
- 1 baked potato, 2 pats of margarine and black pepper (approx. 200 calories)
- 1 salad: 1/2 cup romaine lettuce, 1 raw carrot sliced, 1 tomato sliced, 2 tablespoons vinaigrette dressing (approx. 60 calories)
- 6-ounce grilled flounder seasoned with black pepper and cayenne (approx. 150 calories)
- two 8-ounce glasses of water (0 calories)
- 1 fruit smoothie: 1/2 cup of orange juice, 1 banana, 1/3 cup strawberries (approx. 170 calories)

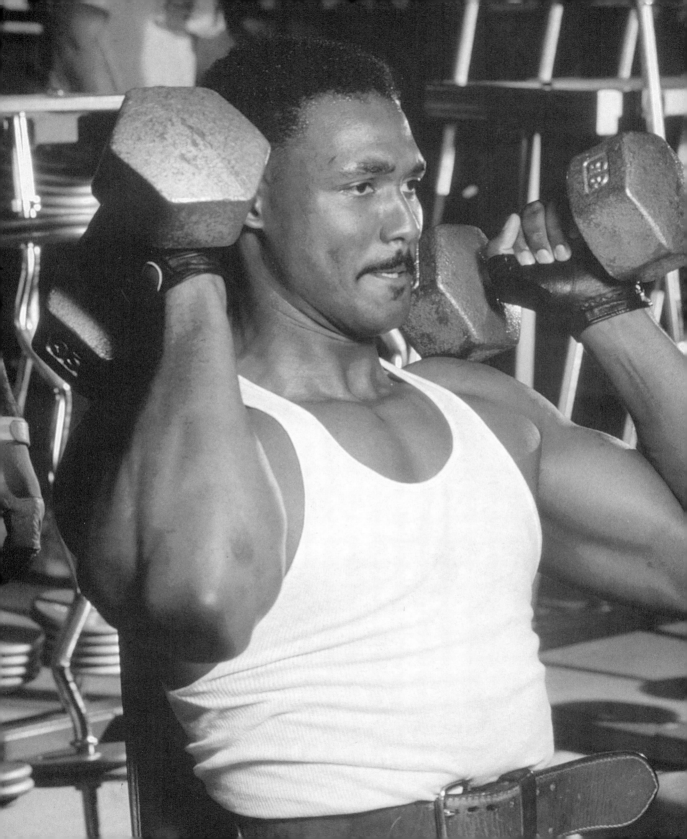

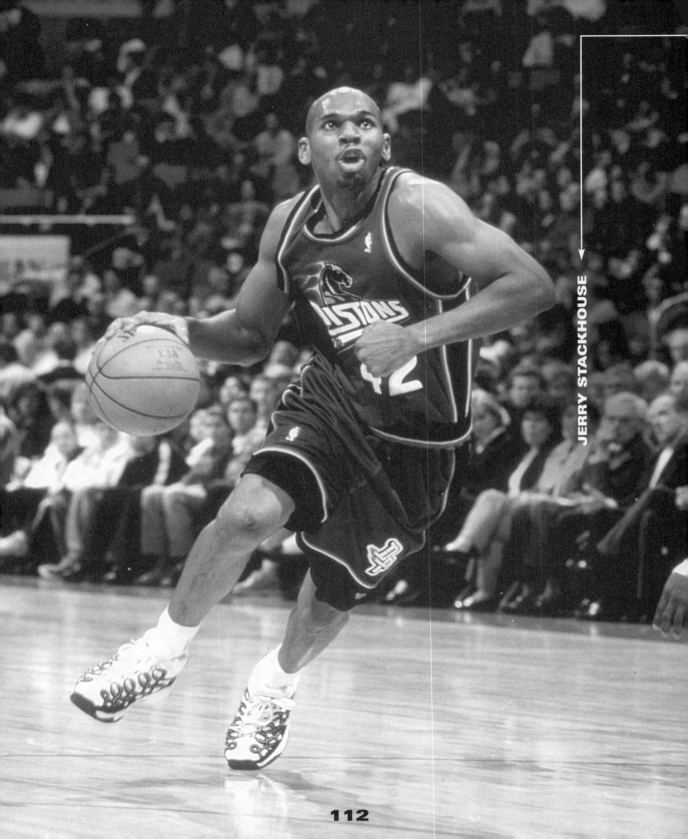

JERRY STACKHOUSE

Most players have their pregame rituals and superstitions. Some of those include what they eat before games. Here is a brief sampling of what an NBA player might ingest before a game, not all of it, by any means, endorsed by the team's trainers.

LaPhonso Ellis, Atlanta Hawks. For home games: peanut butter and spreadable fruit sandwich. On the road: grilled chicken sandwich with lettuce and tomato, an apple and a banana.

Dee Brown, Toronto Raptors: spaghetti.

Hersey Hawkins, Chicago Bulls: pasta.

Scottie Pippen, Portland Trail Blazers: steak and potatoes.

Wesley Person, Cleveland Cavaliers: Reese's Peanut Butter bar or a Kit Kat candy bar.

Jerry Stackhouse, Detroit Pistons: gummy bears.

To Avoid Excess Fat in Your Diet . . .

- Eat lean meat, fish, poultry, peas and dry beans
- Drink low-fat or skim milk
- Limit organ meats and eggs
- Use very small portions of butter, shortening, lard, and certain oils
- Bake, boil, or broil food instead of frying
- Trim fat off meats before cooking them

The Ramadan Diet

Shareef Abdur-Rahim of the Vancouver Grizzlies and Hakeem Olajuwon of the Houston Rockets are both devout Muslims. During the middle of each NBA season is the Muslim holy month of Ramadan, which requires fasting during the daylight hours. That can be tough when trying to perform to the demands of a very hectic NBA schedule. But for both players the sacrifice is worth it. "This is far more important than basketball," says Abdur-Rahim. "This is a time when I'm more at peace with myself and try to get more in touch with God."

Abdur-Rahim's Ramadan schedule includes rising before sunup to eat a breakfast of oatmeal, toast, and a liter of fresh fruit juices. He doesn't eat again until five P.M., two and half hours before tip-off, when he has a light lunch. And after the game he eats his dinner.

"We told him to eat foods that are high in carbohydrates like pasta, grains, and breads," says Grizzlies trainer Troy Wenzel. "We also wanted him to be careful to avoid dehydration."

SHAREEF ABDUR-RAHIM

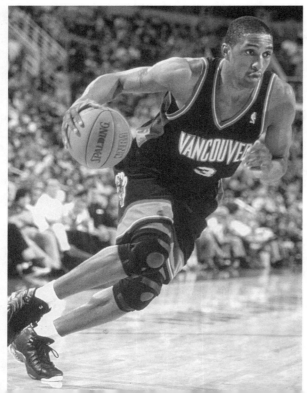

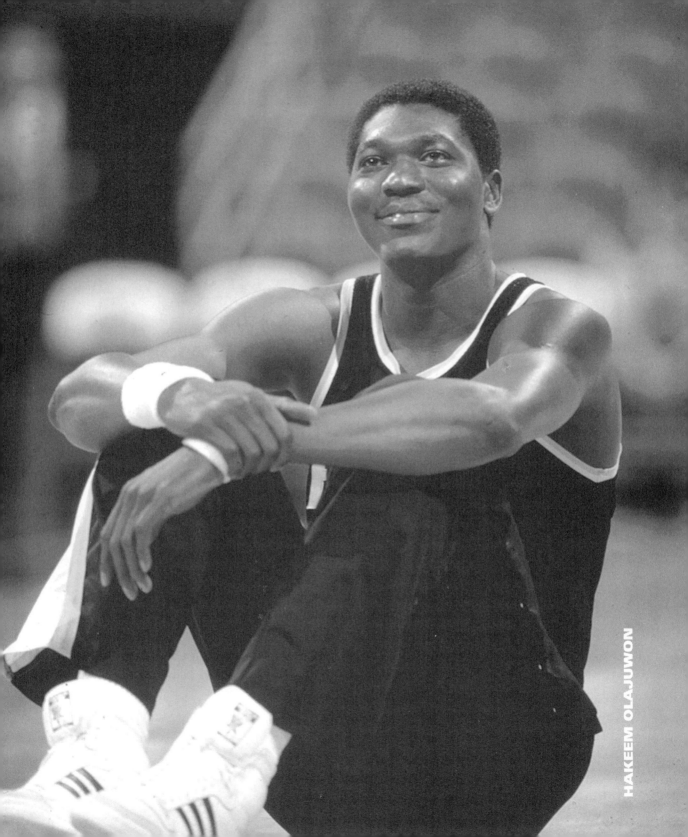

HAKEEM OLAJUWON

The Most Important

Think of any cereal commercial you've ever seen. Isn't the featured bowl always "part of this complete breakfast"? Indeed, just about any nutrition expert will tell you breakfast is the most important meal of the day. Hinds agrees.

"I know some athletes who skip breakfast regularly," Hinds says, "usually with the excuse that they didn't have time or they're not hungry in the morning. As a result, they often have problems concentrating and are irritable. Then, to make up for the lack of breakfast, they eat a big lunch, which leaves them feeling bloated and tired. Don't get into that habit if you expect to benefit from good nutrition. A good, solid breakfast is very important."

Hinds suggests choices such as cereal, oatmeal, milk, a banana, English muffins with jelly, yogurt, whole-grain toast, and orange juice. Choose cereals rich in fiber, bran, iron and calcium, and low in fat and cholesterol. And he advises you to "check the vitamin content of the cereal box while you're at it."

Roger Hinds's ← "Jump Start Breakfast"

- fruit shake consisting of 1/4 of any melon—water, cantaloupe or honeydew—a medium-sized banana, and 6 ounces of fruit juice, all mixed in a blender
- cereal, such as Raisin Bran, All-Bran, or Grape Nuts, or one of the following: whole wheat pancakes or waffles; whole wheat breads; bran muffins
- turkey sausage or turkey bacon (2 links or strips), or one of the following: large glass of milk (if no cereal), 2 scrambled eggs (but no more than three times a week)
- large glass of water

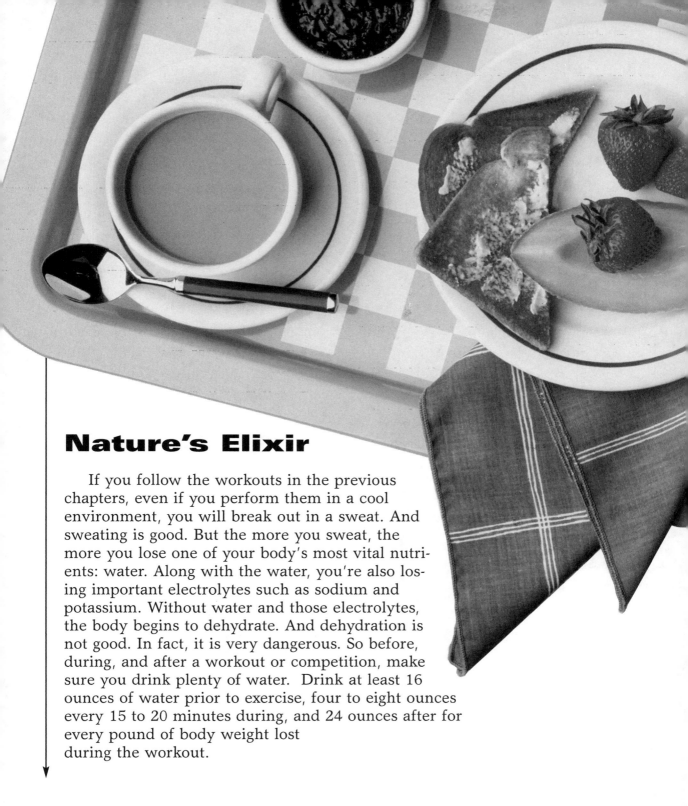

Nature's Elixir

If you follow the workouts in the previous chapters, even if you perform them in a cool environment, you will break out in a sweat. And sweating is good. But the more you sweat, the more you lose one of your body's most vital nutrients: water. Along with the water, you're also losing important electrolytes such as sodium and potassium. Without water and those electrolytes, the body begins to dehydrate. And dehydration is not good. In fact, it is very dangerous. So before, during, and after a workout or competition, make sure you drink plenty of water. Drink at least 16 ounces of water prior to exercise, four to eight ounces every 15 to 20 minutes during, and 24 ounces after for every pound of body weight lost during the workout.

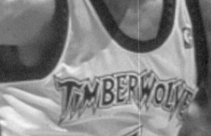

ANTHONY PEELER

Hold the Red Meat

In 1994, Anthony Peeler, then with the Los Angeles Lakers, cut red meat from his diet and switched to fish, chicken, and lots of vegetables.

"Growing up in Kansas City, my mother prepared lots of deep fried foods," says Peeler. "When I was younger I was really chunky. Food was a family thing, and most of the meals were heavy in red meat. I'd feel so full sometimes I'd fall asleep after eating. So I switched. It helped me feel a lot better. It helped me play basketball better too."

Creatine, Energy Bars, and Other Magic Potions

It has hit mainstream America in its collective solar plexus. Walk past the nutrition store in your local mall, and you can't avoid seeing the huge signs featuring huge human beings urging you to bulk up—while laying your money down—for creatine, the most popular of a group of work-enhancing aids known as ergogenic aids.

Thanks to the accomplishments of such athletes as Mark McGwire, creatine and other ergogenic aids have secured a place in the national consciousness. But many athletes are quick to indulge in creatine without really understanding the science behind it.

Creatine is a muscle fuel found in meat and fish, and is produced naturally by your liver. It then travels through your blood to your heart, body cells, and skeletal muscles, where it then forms creatine phosphate, a chemical that supplies energy for muscles, allowing an athlete to perform high intensity, explosive exercises for short periods of time.

There are conflicting opinions on the value and safety of creatine, but Roger Hinds is a proponent of the product, citing its effectiveness and its lack of side effects if

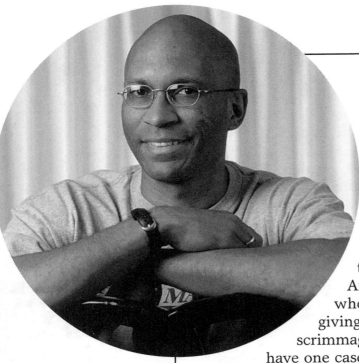

taken in the right dosages. He has used it himself, and found it gave him more intensity in his workouts and sped up his recovery.

"We were administering it to our players last year in tablet form, well below the prescribed doses," Hinds says. "After a loading-up period, we'd give them three grams a day, rather than the five that was recommended. And we only gave it to them on days when we'd do weight training. We'd avoid giving it to them on days when we were scrimmaging or on game days. And we didn't have one case of a serious reaction to it.

"We were looking for recovery from workouts, but that goes along with a good diet. If you're not eating right, it doesn't matter how much creatine you take. It's not a magic pill. It's all a combination. But if you use it the right way, the stuff works. And I don't push it on the players either. A lot of guys ask for it, and we make it available to them if they want to use it."

Still, there are differing viewpoints, even among fellow NBA trainers.

Atlanta Hawks trainer Chris Tucker says, "I've read a lot about the pros and cons of creatine, and while I'm not completely against it, I think athletes have to be very careful about using it. There are too many people taking more than the recommended levels, and the bottom line is that there is not enough research to tell us what's going to happen in ten years to the people who are doing that."

Long-term effects of creatine have not yet been documented, because it is a relatively new ergogenic aid. Large doses have been said to cause muscle tears and gastrointestinal problems, but there is no scentific data to back such claims. The best advice would seem to be common sense. If you do choose to use creatine, consult your physician, consider the opinions of the experts,

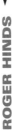

ROGER HINDS

120

don't exceed the recommended dosages, and ignore that muscle-bound cardboard cutout whose best workout regimen is lifting money out of your wallet.

Energy bars and sports beverages can be beneficial to athletes who require replenishing during and after physical activities. These carbohydrate boosts are not just necessary for endurance athletes, as once believed. High intensity exercise can also deplete glycogen stores.

"Some athletes prefer the solid food the energy bar provides, while others like to stick with the sports drinks," says Hinds. "I believe they work well in tandem, and would recommend both if your body can handle them."

Energy bars typically contain between 200 and 300 calories and are 70 to 80 percent carbohydrates, 15 to 20 percent protein, and the remainder fat. Take a pass on bars that contain more than 15 percent fat. Eat an energy bar before you're hungry, and drink fluids with them, such as water or a sports drink.

"Some athletes prefer the solid food the energy bar provides, while others like to stick with the sports drinks," says Hinds.

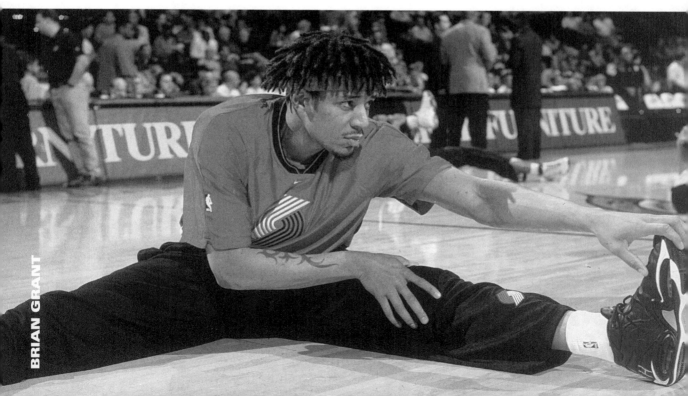

BRIAN GRANT

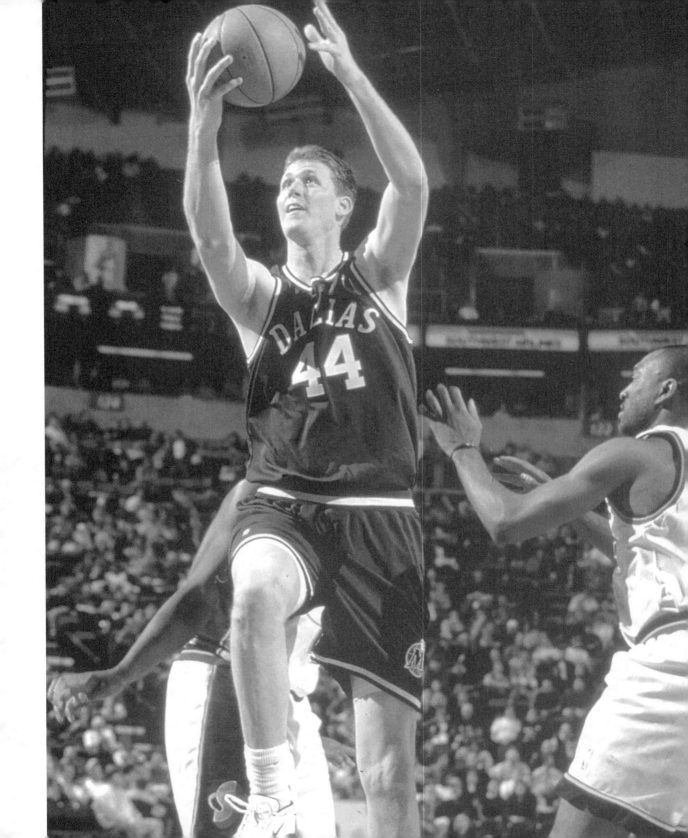

The Bulking of Shawn Bradley

Roger Hinds remembers picking up a copy of *USA Today* one day during the 1994–95 season and leafing through the sports section, as he normally does. Catching his eye was a photo of a bodybuilder, and Hinds, who was the strength and conditioning coach for the Atlanta Hawks at the time, was naturally drawn to it.

And just as naturally, Hinds then had to pick up his jaw, which had fallen to the floor. For superimposed on the bodybuilder was the face of Shawn Bradley, the seven-foot-six center of the Philadelphia 76ers, who had tried almost every method imaginable to put some pounds on his gangly frame.

Hinds had no way of knowing it then, but as head athletic trainer of the Dallas Mavericks, he would one day have his chance to beef up Bradley where others had failed. On the night of Frebruary 17, 1997, Dallas pulled off a nine-player blockbuster trade with the New Jersey Nets, and Bradley became a Maverick.

Just as quickly, Hinds and the Mavericks were presented with a major challenge: How would they succeed in adding weight to Bradley's 248-pound physique?

The panacea was not magic, but good old-fashioned nutrition.

"With Shawn," Hinds says, "we wanted to try to adjust his caloric intake, to give him a positive level, to have more calories stored than he used. We wanted to do it with high carbohydrates, lean meats, and a low-fat diet, which would enable him to gain as much muscle mass as possible.

"And, fortunately for us, when we got Shawn, we had Mother Nature working for us too. Shawn was in his mid-twenties, at the age when his body was at its peak development phase. So, with weight training and paying close attention to what he was eating, when he came back in September 1998, he was thirty pounds heavier than when he left us in April. There was no way he could have done that without his natural growth phase. We just added to it."

"With Shawn, we wanted to try to adjust his calorie intake, to give him a positive level, to have more calories stored than he used. We wanted to do it with high carbohydrates, lean meats, and a low-fat diet, which would enable him to gain as much muscle mass as possible."
Roger Hinds, Athletic Trainer for the Dallas Mavericks

123

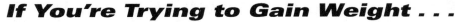

If You're Trying to Gain Weight . . .

A good high-calorie "between meal" meal is Susan Kleiner's High-Calorie Formula from her 1996 book, *High Performance Nutrition—The Total Eating Plan to Maximize Your Workout.* Mix the following in a blender for a great liquid meal:

- 8 ounces of skim milk
- 1 package of instant breakfast
- 1 banana
- 1 tablespoon of peanut butter

The Food Guide Pyramid

The pyramid calls for eating a variety of foods to acquire the nutrients you need, and at the same time the right amount of calories to maintain a healthy weight.

The following daily consumption is recommended:

- 2–3 servings of milk, yogurt, and the cheese group
- 2–3 servings of the meat, poultry, fish, dry beans, eggs, and nuts group
- 3–5 servings of the vegetable group
- 2–4 servings of the fruit group
- 6–11 servings of the bread, cereal, rice, and pasta group
- use fats, oils, and sweets sparingly

Fresh Fruit 4, Doughnuts 0

In the Knicks locker room during the 1999 playoffs vs. the Atlanta Hawks, the Knicks kept the refrigerator stocked with low-fat muffins, fresh fruit, and power bars. At the Hawks training table were boxes of Krispy Kreme dough-nuts. Guess who won the series? See score above.

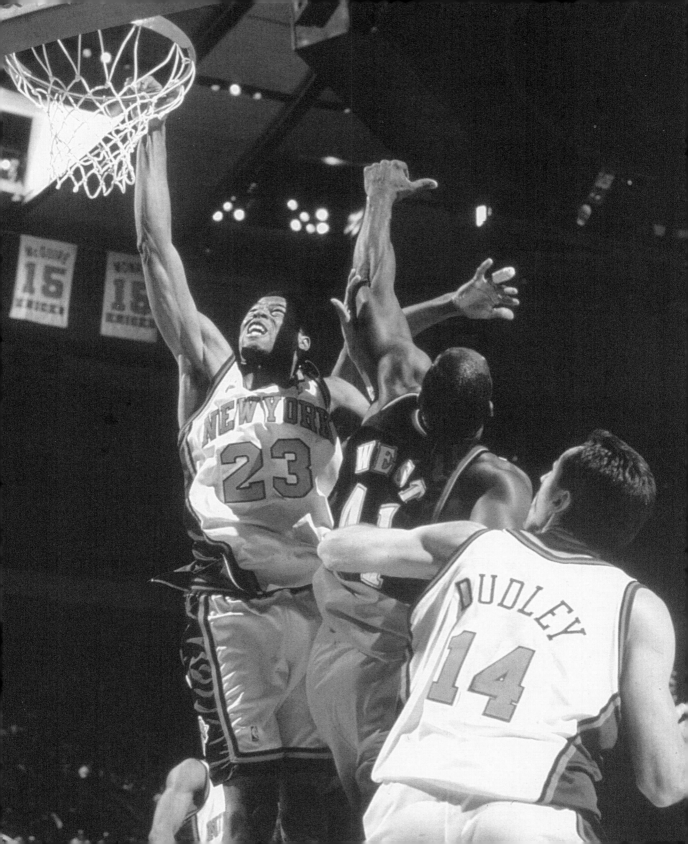

References

Chapter 1

Alter, Judy. *Stretch & Strengthen*. Houghton Mifflin Company, 1986.

Anderson, Bob. *Stretching*. Shelter Publications, Inc., 1980.

Baechle, Thomas R., ed. *Essentials of Strength Training and Conditioning*. National Strength and Conditioning Association, Human Kinetics, 1994.

Foran, Bill. *Condition the NBA Way*. Cadell & Davies (Multi Media Communicators, Inc.), 1994.

Foran, Bill. *NBA Power Conditioning*. National Basketball Conditioning Coaches Association, Human Kinetics, 1997.

Franks, B. Don, and Edward T. Howley. *Fitness Facts—The Healthy Living Handbook*. Human Kinetics, 1989.

Kurz, Thomas. *Stretching Scientifically—A Guide to Flexibility Training*. Stadion Publishing Company, 1994.

Chapter 2

Baechle, Thomas R., ed. *Essentials of Strength Training and Conditioning*. National Strength and Conditioning Association, Human Kinetics, 1994.

Edwards, Sally. *The Heart Rate Monitor Book*. Fleet Feet Press, 1993.

Foran, Bill. *Condition the NBA Way*. Cadell & Davies (Multi Media Communicators, Inc.), 1994.

Foran, Bill. *NBA Power Conditioning*. National Basketball Conditioning Coaches Association, Human Kinetics, 1997.

Franks, B. Don, and Edward T. Howley. *Fitness Facts—The Healthy Living Handbook*. Human Kinetics, 1989.

Janssen, Peter. *Training Lactate Pulse Rate*. Polar Electro Oy, 1987.

Smith, Kathy. *The Ultimate Workout*. Bantam Books, 1983.

Sorensen, Jacki. *Jacki Sorensen's Aerobic Lifestyle Book*. Poseidon Press, 1983.

Staff. *Esquire Ultimate Fitness*. Esquire Press, 1984.

Wilmore, Jack H., and David L. Costill. *Training for Sport and Activity*. William C. Brown Publishers, 1988.

Chapter 3

Baechle, Thomas R., ed. *Essentials of Strength Training and Conditioning.* National Strength and Conditioning Association, Human Kinetics, 1994.

Baechle, Thomas R., and Barney R. Groves. *Weight Training—Steps to Success.* Human Kinetics, 1998.

Brzycki, Matt. *A Practical Approach to Strength Training.* Masters Press, 1995.

Foran, Bill. *Condition the NBA Way.* Cadell & Davies (Multi Media Communicators, Inc.), 1994.

Foran, Bill. *NBA Power Conditioning.* National Basketball Conditioning Coaches Association, Human Kinetics, 1997.

Franks, B. Don, and Edward T. Howley. *Fitness Facts—The Healthy Living Handbook.* Human Kinetics, 1989.

Satterwhite, Yvonne, et al. *Strength and Conditioning Programs: Answers from the Experts* (pamphlet). Sports Science Exchange, 1996.

Chapter 4

Baechle, Thomas R., ed. *Essentials of Strength Training and Conditioning.* National Strength and Conditioning Association, Human Kinetics, 1994.

Baechle, Thomas R. and Barney R. Groves. *Weight Training—Steps to Success.* Human Kinetics, 1998.

Brzycki, Matt. *A Practical Approach to Strength Training.* Masters Press, 1995.

Foran, Bill. *Condition the NBA Way.* Cadell & Davies (Multi Media Communicators, Inc.), 1994.

Foran, Bill. *NBA Power Conditioning.* National Basketball Conditioning Coaches Association, Human Kinetics, 1997.

Franks, B. Don, and Edward T. Howley. *Fitness Facts—The Healthy Living Handbook.* Human Kinetics, 1989.

Micheli, Lyle J., M.D. *The Sports Medicine Bible.* HarperPerennial (HarperCollins Publishers), 1995.

Satterwhite, Yvonne, et al. (pamphlet); Sports Science *Strength and Conditioning Programs: Answers from the Experts.* Sports Science Exchange, 1996.

Williams, J.P.R. *Barron's Sports Injury Handbook.* Amanuensis

Books Limited, 1988.

Chapter 5

Baechle, Thomas R., ed. *Essentials of Strength Training and Conditioning.* National Strength and Conditioning Association, Human Kinetics, 1994.

Burke, Edmund R., and Jacqueline R. Berning. *Training Nutrition— The Diet and Nutrition Guide for Peak Performance.* Cooper Publishing Group, 1996.

Clark, Nancy. *Nancy Clark's Sports Nutrition Guidebook.* Human Kinetics, 1997.

Foran, Bill. *Condition the NBA Way.* Cadell & Davies (Multi Media Communicators, Inc.), 1994.

Foran, Bill. *NBA Power Conditioning; National Basketball Conditioning Coaches Association.* Human Kinetics, 1997.

Franks, B. Don, and Edward T. Howley. *Fitness Facts—The Healthy Living Handbook.* Human Kinetics, 1989.

Kleiner, Susan. *High Performance Nutrition—The Total Eating Plan to Maximize Your Workout.* John Wiley & Sons, 1996.

Staff. *You Are What You Eat. The NutraSense Journal,* The NutraSense Company, 1998.

Biography

Timothy Boyle has 23 years of professional writing experience. A former news writer and sports editor for the *Suburban Life Graphic* newspaper in Downers Grove, Illinois, and a freelance sportswriter for the *Daily Herald* newspaper of Arlington Heights, Illinois, Boyle co-authored *Baseball's Best: The MVPs* (Contemporary Books, Inc., 1985). He has also written numerous freelance articles for a variety of magazines and newspapers.

Boyle owns and operates Double M Communications, a small public relations firm, out of Kenosha, Wisconsin, where he resides with wife, Deanna, daughter, Kaitlyn, and stepsons, Jon and Tyler. Boyle graduated from Northern Illinois University with a bachelor of science degree in 1976.